Red Jungle Fowl

RED JUNGLE FOWL

Edited by :

DEEPAK SHARMA

Ph.D., Principal Scientist & Head

Division of Animal Genetics, Indian Veterinary Research Institute, Izatnagar 243 122 (UP)

SSPH

SATISH SERIAL PUBLISHING HOUSE

403, Express Tower, Commercial Complex
Azadpur, Delhi-110033 (India)
Phone : 011-27672852, Fax : 91-11-27672046
E-mail : info@satishserial.com,
hkjain1975@yahoo.com
Website : www.satishserial.com

Published by :

SATISH SERIAL PUBLISHING HOUSE

403, Express Tower, Commercial Complex, Azadpur,
Delhi-110033 (INDIA)
Phone : 011-27672852 Fax : 91-11-27672046
E-mail : info@satishserial.com,
hkjain1975@yahoo.com

ISBN 978-93-81226-47-6

Typeset at: Harminder Kharb *for* Laxmi Art Creation
Printed at: Salasar Imaging Systems, Delhi-110035

Contents

Preface

Chicken egg and meat is among one of the important source of human food. Chicken egg is considered as cheapest source of high quality animal protein. Chicken farming has taken a shape of an organized commercial sector and India has a strong standing globally being third highest egg producer and fifth highest broiler producer. Presently, global poultry industry is a multi-multimillion dollar Industry.

Domestication of chicken dates back to 5000 BC. Chicken was domesticated for religious activities, decorative arts, and entertainment initially and much later it was started to be utilized as human food. Development of highly specialized lines of chicken of egg and meat type started in 19th century only. Presently, egg type chicken lays more than 330 eggs in a year and meat type chicken weights more than one kg in 30-35 days. This process of manmade selection has changed the chicken genome and in the process, some attributes might have lost, while some has gained. The red jungle fowl is believed to be the ancestor of all the to-days chicken and have its existence to-days also. Hence the comparative genomic analysis will help the scientists in understanding the gains and losses at genetic levels, occurred in the process of transformation of chicken to a egg and meat producing machine.

Present book deals with the overview of the distribution and physical appearance of the different species of jungle fowls including subspecies of Red jungle fowl, early history of domestication and origin of domestic chicken, while later chapters covers the molecular characterization of India Red Jungle fowl. I hope that this book will be of great help to the students as well as academicians.

(Deepak Sharma)

Introduction

The domestic chicken is among the most popular and widely spread domestic animal species. For thousand years, chickens have been used for food, religious activities, decorative arts and entertainment. In present time chicken rearing has taken a shape of industry. Presently, global annual broiler meat production is more than 80 million tonnes and egg production is more than 120 million tonnes. It makes the global poultry industry a multi-multimillion dollar Industry. Poultry industry in India has a strong standing globally, being third highest egg producer with more than 54000 million eggs and fifth highest broiler producer with 2.25 million tones of broiler meat. Largely, Indian poultry industry is chicken dominated and the rearing of high yielding varieties under intensive rearing system is the back bone of its present face.

The evolution of chicken can be conceived as a three step process- evolution and speciation of wild ancestor, domestication of wild species and diversification toward development of different breeds. There are four known species of jungle fowls and are known as Red jungle fowl, Grey jungle fowl, Green jungle fowl and Ceylon jungle fowl. All the jungle fowls are found in Southeast Asia. While the Ceylon jungle fowl and green jungle fowls are native of Sri Lanka and Java, respectively, Grey jungle fowl is native of southern and western India. There are five subspecies of red jungle fowls and all have their respective native tracks i.e. *G. g. gallus* in Thailand and its adjacent regions, *G. g. spadiceus* in Burma and Yunnan Province of China and northeast part of India, *G. g. jabouillei* in southern China and Vietnam, *G. g. murghi* in India and *G. g. bankiva* in the Java islands.

Among the four jungle fowls Red jungle fowl is considered as the sole ancestor of the domestic chicken. There are various morphological, biochemical and genetical including molecular evidences to support this most favored theory, however in view of certain evidences coming from possible mating between domestic chicken and other jungle fowls and also some genetical evidences, the possibilities of contributions from other jungle fowl may be possible. But apart from these arguments-counter arguments, the Indian red jungle fowl does not lose its importance of being sole/major ancestor in view of the strong evidences of domestication in Indus valley (2000-2500 BC).

As per view of some researchers, the Indian red jungle fowl is facing a danger of extinction, especially in terms of the quality (Peterson and Brisbin, 1999), while other believes that these threats are not real and the Indian RJF is genetically pure (Kanginakudru et al., 2008). Hence there is need to characterize the Indian RJF genetically for various aspects at molecular level. The present book is an initiation in this direction. First four chapters of this book present the overview of the distribution and physical appearance of the different species of jungle fowls including subspecies of Red jungle fowl, early history of domestication and origin of domestic chicken, while later chapters covers the molecular characterization of India Red Jungle fowl.

❑❑❑

Chapter 1

History of Domestication of Chicken

The question of domestication of chicken is still debatable. Earlier, in majority of reviews, the Indus valley is considered as the point of first domestication in 2500-2100 BC, however, later, much earlier domestication of chicken in Southeast Asia and than in china (~5000 BC) was evidenced. In early reviews, the opinion of Peters (1913) did not get enough consideration as his statements lacked literary and/or archaeological evidences. Though, Darwin (1896) expressed a similar belief and West and Zhou (1988) have provided strong evidences in support of later theory. However, the evidences of domestication of chicken at two different places in two different times are unquestionable and they are Harappan culture of Indus valley (2500-2100 BC) and ancient china (> 5400 BC).

The Harappan culture dates back to 2500-2100 BC and was the first urban civilization on the Indian subcontinent. It occupied a huge area of the Indus valley and plain in present-day Pakistan. The twin capital cities of Harappa and Mohenjo-Daro are the best known archaeological sites. Agriculture was the economic base for the Harappan culture, and there was an extensive trade network with Sumeria and Mesopotamia. The evidences for domestication of chicken were the seals found at Mohenjo-Daro depicting fighting cocks, clay collectibles of chickens including one of a hen with a feed dish, chicken bones (Femur ~ 130 mm in size) which was much larger than that of jungle fowl (~ 69 mm) suggesting positive selection for body size. Zeuner (1963) estimated that domestication of chickens was complete by about 2000 BC, however Wood-Gush (1959, 1985) predicted it to be 3200 BC, though his predictions were not based on the evidences from Harrapan and Mohan jo daro remnants.

There are several discoveries and supporting evidences of chicken domestication in ancient China, which indicate that domestic fowl was domesticated much earlier than the Indus valley culture i.e. as early as 5400 BC. Short descriptions of some discoveries have been given by Ho (1977) and Watson (1969). Plant (1985) has reviewed and reprinted an English translation of parts of a 1981 paper by Zhou Ben-Xiong (also known as Chow Ben-Shun) concerning discoveries at the Cishan site. Chow (1984) has published an English-language review of the discoveries, and they have also been reviewed by West and Zhou (1988). From the archaeological site of Cishan, in Wu'an county of Hebei province, the chicken remains were found and most of them were tarsometatarsal bones (from males as well as females). Among other bones, clavicle, humerus, femur and radius and ulna specimens were also found. These chicken bones were in abundance in the animal remains and the much larger size of these bones in comparison to that of red jungle fowl reveal positive evidence for domestication (Zhou, 1981, in Plant, 1985). During the same time period, similar bone discoveries were also made at the Pei-li-Kang site in Henan province (Chow, 1984). Chow's (1984) interpreted that chicken domestication may have occurred as early as 6000 BC. Evidences of chicken domestications were also found during Yang Shao culture of south Shensi, which dates back to 4800-3000 BC.

West and Zhou (1988) reviewed several evidences and found that 16 Neolithic sites in northern China have now yielded evidence of domestic fowl, all of them predating Mohenjo-Daro by many centuries. At 13 sites in Europe and western Asia, chicken bones older than those of Mohenjo-Daro were discovered. Eight other sites in China, Turkey, Syria, Spain, Romania, and the Ukraine have yielded osteological evidence that is contemporary with that of Mohenjo-Daro. Further, using information from Ho (1977) and from other sources, West and Zhou (1988) stated that the semiarid climates at the 16 Neolithic sites during at least past 10000 years, was the normal climate for jungle fowl, hence they proposed the domestication point of chicken somewhere in southeast Asia and its subsequent travel to northern China by about 6000 BC. These evidences put the question mark on the Indus valley as the first domestication centre.

Using archaeological evidence for chicken domestication from China, Asia and Europe, as well as palaeo-climatic evidence from China, it is concluded that chickens were first domesticated from the red jungle fowl (*Gallus gallus*) in Southeast Asia well before the sixth millennium BC and taken north to become established in China by 6000 BC, where they were later introduced to Japan via Korea during the Yayoi Period (300 BC-300 AD). Domestication occurred in India much later than that in China (~ 2000 BC), either independently or as a diffusion from Southeast Asia. Although the Iron Age was the main period for dispersion of chickens throughout Europe, they were already present in some areas during the late Neolithic and early Bronze Age. It is proposed that the earliest European material may be derived from China via Russia.

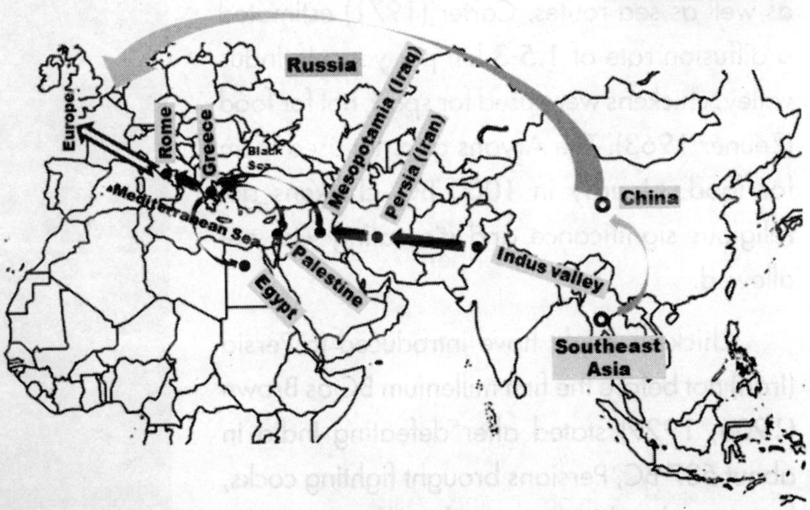

Fig. 1.1 : Diagrammatic representation of possible route(s) of domestic chicken expansion

Westward expansion of chicken

The expansion of chicken has been discussed in all the recent reviews of chicken history (Crawford 1984; Wood-Gush 1959; Zeuner 1963), keeping Indus valley as a point of first domestication and this theory has a strong literally support. However, the existence of chicken at some of the places much earlier than the periods mentioned in this theory cannot be denied in view of the osteological evidences reviewed by West and Zhou (1988). So the most accepted expansion route of the domestication of chicken may be follows.

From the Indus valley, the expansion of the chicken was gradual and might have taken land as well as sea routes. Carter (1971) estimated a diffusion rate of 1.5-3 km per year. In Indus valley, chickens were used for sport, not for food (Zeuner 1963). The Aryans also not used them for food. Nearby in 1000 BC, chickens got religious significance and it's eating was not allowed.

Chickens might have introduced to Persia (Iran) not before the first millenium BC as Brown (1906, 1929) stated after defeating India in about 537 BC, Persians brought fighting cocks, however, the chickens must have been existing much earlier as in Zoroastrian literature of the

Kianian Period (2000-700 BC) the cock was known as the Herald of the Dawn (Wood-Gush, 1959) and it also played a role as guardian of good against evil (Zeuner 1963). The chicken travelled more westward to Mesopotamia and Asia Minor (Zeuner 1963) and Medes were key players for this expansion as chickens has been mentioned as Median bird in Greek reference. Role of chicken in religious activities is evident from the seals belonging to eighth century BC. The cock-fighting remained very popular.

Chicken might have reached to Greece from Persia in seventh century BC as per Pollard (1977). First mention of chicken is by Theogens (ancient Greek Poet) who wrote in the latter half of the sixth century BC. Zeuner (1963) stated that after induction, the chickens were very rapidly accepted and spread wide over up to distant Greek colonies in Sicily and southern Italy. But still chicken were used for sport, apart from their role in religious and cultural activities. Apart from domestication, diversification was also evidenced in during Greek period (Pollard, 1977) and both Plato and Aristotle distinguished between high-bred and low-bred chickens as high bred birds were poor in egg laying. Different breeds such as one, black in colour with crest and wattles 'like anemones' (may be referred as rose comb mutant) and a bearded chicken, might be muffs and beard mutant were known.

In Egypt, under Greek and Persian influence, the chickens were inducted and got strong footing (Coltherd, 1966). Regarding the time period of its induction in Egypt, there are some controversies. There are number of strong evidences, which suggest the existence of chicken between 1200-1500 BC, but after that there is no record of chicken existence till 600 BC.

The evidences regarding the existence of chicken before 1200 BC includes a steatite seal from Crete, dating back to about 1500 BC clearly depicts a rooster (Lowe 1934), representation of a chicken on blocks from a temple of the Middle Kingdom near Thebes, dated at about 1840 BC, and mention of 'four birds of this country' in the "list of tribute from an Asian land" in Royal annals of Thutmose III (1479-1447 BC). Three pictorial evidences i.e. rooster's head in a mural from the tomb of Rekhmara, vizier of Thutmose III (1450 BC), at Thebes, painting of a rooster on an ostracon found in association with the tomb of Tutankhamun and probably contemporary with his burial in 1338 BC and a figure of the roaster on silver bowl from the reign of Seti II (1200-1194 BC) are very strong evidences (Coltherd, 1966). These evidences may represent the existence of foreign trade, rather than rearing of chickens in Crete and Egypt. Egypt faced the political decline and recession in trade in ~ 1000 BC. Till, 600 BC, no mention of the chicken was found and in 600 BC, there are several pictorial and literary records of chicken existence in Egypt.

In Palestine, the existence of chicken was recorded in 7th century, BC and it was used exclusively for fighting sports (Taran, 1975). But the absence of mention of chicken in Old Testament, suggested that chicken did not get entry in Palestine before 200 BC (Wood-Gush, 1959). Peter (1913) also concluded that there is no mention of chicken in Old Testament; however it is frequently mentioned in New Testament.

Romans might have introduced chickens from the Greek colonies in the south of Italy, but a separate route from the north is also possible (Hyams, 1972; Zeuner (1963). By the first century BC, poultry rearing has improved a lot and there are mentions of knowing the force feeding, hybrid vigor, caponizing, and even about sperm competition by Romans (Lind,

1963). They had many breeds or types and they have reared the chicken for food also, apart from cock-fighting sport and in religion, superstition, and divination.

Induction of chickens to Europe north of the Mediterranean is not very well known. There are several opinions. Brown (1929) stated that the chickens might have reached Europe by two routes i.e. via Iran and the Mediterranean or by a northern route across China and Russia in AD 1300. As per Peters (1913), chicken travelled to Europe from Iran, possibly by two routes i.e. via the Aegean Sea to the Greeks and Romans, and via the Black Sea and Scythia reaching central Europe through southern Russia. Carter (1971) supported Peters' two routes, using linguistic evidence as gradual change of the Sanskrit world *pil* from India to *pullet* and *gallus* in Mediterranean and western Europe; and evolution of Sanskrit *kukuta* through central and northern Europe to become *chicken* and *cock.* Bokonyi (1984) opinion of bringing chicken first to Hungary by the Scythians (about 500 BC) favored Peters' second route.

From the work of West and Zhou (1988), it seems that the main period for dispersion through Europe was the Iron Age, but chickens were already present in some areas during the late Neolithic and early Bronze Age. Chickens seemed to be widespread in Europe by the first century BC (Zeuner, 1963) as evident from the getting the bones dating from this period in Switzerland, Germany, and England (Bate, 1934; Harrison 1978), but it is also evident that Romans also carried the chicken with them as the bones have been recovered from a number of Roman sites (Zeuner, 1963).

In popularizing the chicken throughout their empire and secondarily with their spread beyond Roman boundaries, Romans played a significant role, however, chickens were existing earlier across most of Europe. Fall of Roman Empire also resulted in decline in organized and planned poultry rearing throughout Europe, and chickens were being reared as farmyard scavengers (Wood-Gush, 1959). Beginning of the 19th century, the poultry rearing got attention.

In Africa, except for Egypt, little is known about introduction of chickens to Africa. Sauer (1969) said they were already present at the time of first European contact. Chickens with black feathers, meat, and bones were described from Mozambique in 1635. The fibromelanosis mutant was known in India at that time but not in Europe. Carter (1971) showed that words for chickens in both East and West Africa had an Indian root. Origin from India is likely because trade between India and the east coast of Africa was well-developed at an early date.

Eastward expansion of Chicken

The spread of chickens eastward from the Indus valley has received little study. Till date, all the theories regarding expansion of chicken from the point of first domestication are based on the assumption that Indus valley domestication was the first and sole domestication point. But in view of the osteological evidences, summarized by West and Zhou (1988), if it is to be considered that a separate and much earlier domestication occurred in China or if even still more early domestication occurred in Southeast Asia, then the whole expansion theory is to be redefined.

Induction of chicken in America

Existence of chicken in America in Pre-Columbian time received much attention. Jett (1983) overviewed the evidence for pre-Columbian transoceanic contacts. The existence of better watercrafts with Southeast and Southwest Asians suggesting the possible travel to America via Pacific, very strong similarities between Asian and American cultures in architecture, art and decoration, tools and weapons, religious practices, and language are strong evidences. Carter (1971) reviewed biological, cultural, and linguistic evidences, which as strongly suggests introduction of chickens to South America from across the Pacific many centuries before the Spanish Conquest. But conclusive proof from skeletal remains from pre-Columbian sites are lacking. The usual view is that chickens first arrived during the Spanish Conquest and spread rapidly thereafter through South and Central America. Much later the English, French, and Dutch brought them to eastern North America.

□□□

Chapter **2**

Body Parts of Gallus Birds

Body parts of Gallus birds

The genus Gallus includes four species i.e. *Gallus lafayetti, Gallus varius, Gallus sonneratti* and *Gallus gallus.* The domestic chicken is considered as one of the subspecies of *Gallus gallus.* The body parts of a domestic chicken are being depicted and briefly described.

1 **Head:** Comprises of skull, comb, face, eyes, beak, earlobes and wattles

2 **Beak:** Two horny mandibles projecting from the front of face

3 **Wattle:** Flesh appendages at each side of the base of beak

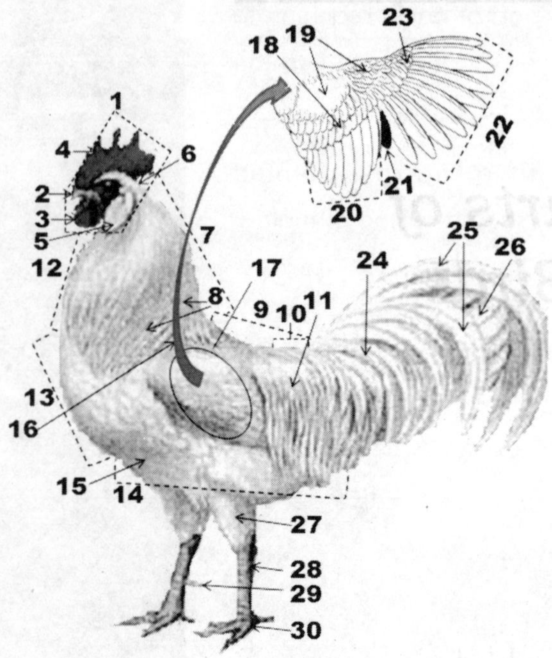

Fig. 2.1 : Common body parts of a male chicken

4 **Comb:** fleshy protuberance on top of the head

5 **Earlobes:** fold of skin hanging below the ears

6 **Crest:** tuft of feathers on head

7 **Neck:** from the base of head to start of back/ breast

8 **Neck hackle:** neck feathers of fowl

9 **Back:** top of the body from base of neck to beginning of tail

1 0 **Saddle:** posterior part of back, reaching to tail of male and corresponding to cushion in female

1 1 **Saddle hackle:** long, narrow pointed feathers present in saddle region of male

1 2 **Throat:** front side of neck

1 3 **Breast:** front of fowl,s body from point of keel to base of neck

1 4 **Abdomen:** under part of body from keel to vent

1 5 **Keel:** blades of keel bone

1 6 **Scapular:** shoulder feathers

1 7 **Wing:** modified forelimbs in birds

1 8 **Lower wing coverts:** feather covering the roots of the secondary quills

1 9 **Upper wing coverts:** feather covering the roots of the secondary quills

2 0 **Secondaries:** quill feather of wings which are visible in closed wings

2 1 **Axial feather:** A feather in wing separating primaries and secondaries

2 2 **Primaries:** flight feathers of wing (10 in numbers), not visible in resting bird

23 **Flight feather:** small stiff feathers covering base of primaries

24 **Tail Coverts:** covering feathers of tail

25 **Sickles:** in general long curved feathers of tail in male

26 **Tail feathers:** straight and stiff feathers of tail only

27 **Thigh:** part of leg above the shank and covered with feathers

28 **Leg:** shank or scaly part

29 **Spur:** horny projection on shank of males, sometime in females

30 **Claw:** foot having four toes

□□□

Chapter 3

Species and Sub Species of Jungle Fowl

In general, Junglefowl refers to the four species of bird under the genus *gallus*, order Galliformes and family Phasianidae. The jungle fowls are large birds with colourful male plumage and dull female plumage. These jungle fowls are found in India, Sri Lanka, Southeast Asia and Indonesia.

Most common name	Zoological name	Other names
Ceylon jungle fowl	*G. lafayetti*	*Gallus Stanleyi* *Gallus lafayetti Lesson*
Green Jungle fowl	*G. varius*	*Gallus varius Shaw*
Grey Jungle fowl	*G. sonneratti*	*Gallus sonnerati Temminck*
Red Jungle fowl	*G. gallus*	*Gallus gallus Linnaeus*

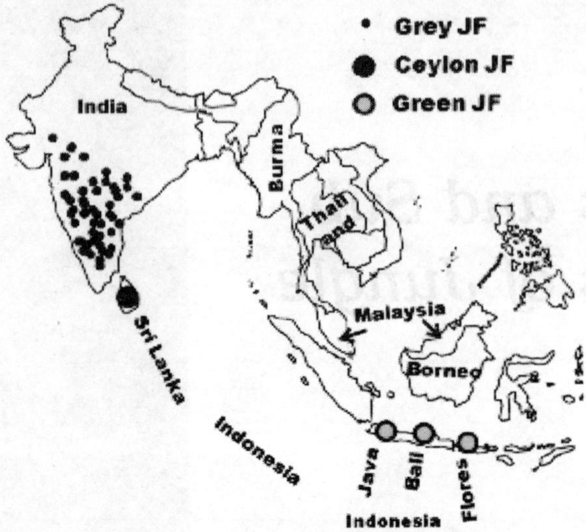

Fig. 3.1 : Distribution of three jungle fowls

Ceylon or Sri Lanka jungle fowl

The Ceylon Junglefowl is native to Sri Lanka, from whence it derives its name; Sri Lanka was once called Ceylon. It is also known as Jungle fowl–Ceylon or Ceylon Jungle fowl. *Gallus lafayettii*, sometimes also named *Gallus Stanleyi*.

Taxonomic classification

Kingdom	Animalia
Phylum	Chordata
Class	Aves
Order	Galliformes
Family	Phasianidae
Genus	Gallus
Species	G. lafayetti

Distribution

This subspecies inhabits exclusively the island of Ceylon (Sri Lanka), both in plane and mountain areas, where it can be found up to 1,700 mt.

Phenotypic Appearance

While most of the body of males is shiny blackish-purple, majority of body covered with brown feather.

Male

Comb: slightly indented and has a spot of bright yellow

Head: bright red, feather less face, wattles-red, beak-brown; iris-yellowish white

Neck: neck hackles – yellow gold coloured sometime red with dark flames in centre of feathers; Undergo molting

Back: feathers bordered in orange

Saddle: purple red at base with a bluish hue at their apex

Rump: red with black stripes

Tail: black with blue sheen.

Breast: yellow gold coloured sometime red with dark flames in centre of feathers.

Abdomen: bright red with fine black stripes

Wing: Wing coverts – orange red central black strip, primeries-blackish brown, secondary wing covert-with blue sheen

Legs: red orange, shank-yellow red

Female

Comb: very tiny comb

Head: feather on face which are brown and small, no wattle

Neck: neck hackles have black patches with yellow accent

Rump: brown

Tail: tail feathers are black, richly speckled with reddish brown

Breast: upper portion is brown and have large tan or cream central lanceolate. Feathers on lower breast are typically white with black and brown feathers interspersed.

Abdomen: white with irregular stripes oand black endings

Wing: secondary wing coverts are black with brown yellowish stripes in the width

Legs: red orange

Javan Junglefowl (Green Jungle fowl)

The Green Jungle fowl, is also known as Javan Jungle fowl, Forktail or Green Javanese Junglefowl.

Taxonomic Classification

Kingdom	Animalia
Phylum	Chordata
Class	Aves
Order	Galliformes
Family	Phasianidae
Genus	Gallus
Species	G. varius

Distribution

This species is originally of Java, but also found in Bali, Lombok, Komodo, Flores, Rinca and Indonesia.

Phenotypic Appearance

Males are mostly green and black feathered, while females are mostly brown.

Male

Comb: Green at base and centre, turning purplish red towards border, have no indentation

Head: Short feathers, black at basis, blue in centre and golden green on remaining surface. Wattle-purplish-red, bordered with blue on edges and yellow nearer the throat, beak-horn coloured, iris-fire red

Neck: Lighter green and blue patterns. It do not go under ecplipse molting.

Saddle: Saddle hackles are dark green with edges of yellow

Rump: Upper part of rump have feathers, black at basis, blue in centre and golden green on remaining surface, while lower part have golden green with blue sheen.

Tail: Held low black, with a light greenish blue shade

Breast: Black, also with a light greenish blue shade

Abdomen: Black, also with a light greenish blue shade

Wing: Primaries and primary coverts- black with a slight greenish blue shade, Lower and middle wing coverts- long in shape, red orange in color with a long central black stripe;

Legs: Flesh coloured shank

Female

Comb: Absent

Head: Head- brown, with black stripes, face sides-light brown, wattle-scarcely developed

Neck: Jet brown, with black stripes, thorat-white

Back: Black with irregular yellowish strips

Tail: Black with irregular brown spots

Breast: Black with irregular yellowish strips

Abdomen: Leather coloured

Wing: Primaries and primary wing coverts=dark brown; Secondaries and secondary wing coverts- black with irregular yellowish strips

Grey Junglefowl

Grey Junglefowl, also known as Sonnerat's Junglefowl and this name commemorates the French explorer Pierre Sonnerat.

Taxonomic Classification

Kingdom	Animalia
Phylum	Chordata
Class	Aves
Order	Galliformes
Family	Phasianidae
Genus	Gallus
Species	G. sonneratti

Distribution

Indigenous to Southern and Western India, but extends into Gujarat, Madhya Pradesh and south Rajasthan. This species and the Red Junglefowl overlap slightly along the northern boundary of the distributio although the ranges are largely non-overlapping.

Phenotypic Appearance

Main characteristic of this fowl is the extraordinary dilation of the apical part of the shaft, or rachis in the neck and saddle hackles, and the tail coverts. Through this dilation, these feathers seem covered with scales, which confers them a very different look.

Male

Comb: Small, red with slight indentation

Head: Red earlobes, horn-coloured beak, on head, black feathers showing grey fringes and a white bar and a straw-yellow stain in the terminal part

Neck: Neck hackle- black, with grey fringes and a white bar and a straw-yellow stain in the terminal part. Scapulars- black, with a white yellowish stripe along the shaft that expands towards the apex in a wide orange spot with external red fringes. Neck feathers undergo eclipse plumage.

Saddle: Main saddle feathers- show orange and red fringes and are embellished with yellow flame-shaped spots in the apex; remaining part of the saddle are purple shaded, with a grey edging and a thin white stripe along the shaft;

Rump: Feathers on the forepart of the rump - are black, with grey fringes, a white bar and a straw-yellow stain in the terminal part, while remaining part of the rump, are purple shaded, with a grey edging and a thin white stripe along the shaft.

Tail: Tail, black with purple sheen. Central tail feathers long and sickle shaped.

Breast: Grey colour

Abdomen: Abdomen and lower parts of the body is grey.

Wing: Primaries and primary coverts, brown-black.

Legs: Shanks- deep orange yellow with spur.

Female

Comb: Comb is extremely small and dull red,

Head: Brown with light streaks on forehead and most of the part of face is feathered.

Neck: Feathers display white yellowish stripes along the shaft

Back: Feathers are mottled brown and black

Rump: Feathers are mottled brown and black and display white yellowish stripes along the shaft.

Breast: White

Abdomen: Light buff

Wing: Feathers- mottled brown and black

Red Junglefowl

The red jungle fowl (RJF) is largest species among jungle fowl as five different subspecies have been identified.

Common name	Zoological name	Other names
Cochin-Chinese RJF	*G. gallus gallus*	*Gallus gallus gallus Linnaeus*
Indian RJF	*G. gallus murghi*	*Gallus gallus murghi Robinson & Kloss*
Burmese RJF	*G. gallus spadiceus*	*Gallus gallus spadiceus Bonnaterre*
Tonkinese RJF	*G gallus jabouillei*	*Gallus g. jabouillei Delacoure Kinnea*
Javan RJF	*G. gallus bankiva*	*Gallus gallus bankiva Temminck* *Gallus gallus ferrugineus Gmelin*

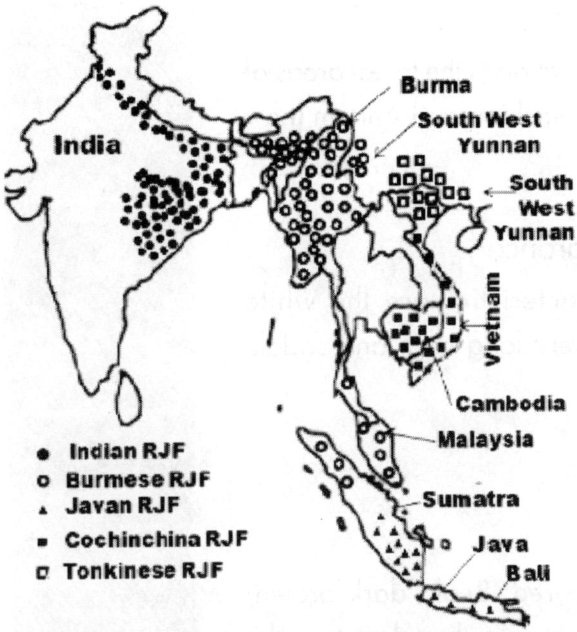

Fig. 3.2 : Distribution of five subspecies of Red Jungle fowl

Cochin-Chinese red jungle fowl

Taxonomic Classification

Kingdom	Animalia
Phylum	Chordata
Class	Aves
Order	Galliformes
Family	Phasianidae
Genus	Gallus
Species	G. gallus
Sub-species	G. g. gallus

Distribution

This subspecies inhabits the forest areas of Cambodia and Cochinchina and Annam (now Vietnam).

Phenotypic Appearance

Its main characteristics are the white earlobes, and the very long neck and saddle hackles.

Male

Comb: red

Head: Wattles- red; Beak- dark brown; white earlobes, other non-feathered parts on the head and neck, red;

Neck: Dark orange or orange red coloured, turning orange and deep yellow on the tips of the longest neck feathers, Scapulars- dark brown red, turning into deep orange

During the summer molt, the black and tan striped hackles and lanceolates or neck hackles are replaced by regularly shaped, hen-like feathers, of a jet black colour. The hackles grow again in the autumn.

Back: Back are dark brown red, turning into deep orange on the long sharp saddle hackles

Rump: Black with a green or purple blue sheen

Tail: Main upper tail coverts and tail, black with green and purple blue sheen with a white tuft at base.

Abdomen: Abdomen and lower part of the body black with green sheen

Wing: Secondaries and primary wing coverts are black with a green or purple blue sheen, middle wing coverts are dark brown red. Remiges- black, with a brown external edging in the primaries, while the external half of the vane (i.e., the barbs considered collectively as a flat surface) is chestnut or brown red;

Legs: slate grey shanks.

Female

Comb: Very tiny

Head: Yellow

Neck: Neck hackle- yellow with black flames in length, scapulars- uniform brownish colour which is black-pencilled, with a neat, deep golden lacing. The rachis or shaft is whitish yellow.

Back: Uniform brownish colour which is black-pencilled, with a neat, deep golden lacing. The rachis or shaft is whitish yellow.

Tail: Black and brown pencilled

Breast: Light salmon colour

Abdomen: Ash brown with finely edged feathers

Wing: Primaries- slate brown, the outer barbs showing a thin brown edging/brim, Secondary wing coverts or remiges- brown, with finely pencilled light brown barbs.

Indian red jungle fowl

Taxonomic Classification

Kingdom	Animalia
Phylum	Chordata
Class	Aves
Order	Galliformes
Family	Phasianidae
Genus	Gallus
Species	G. gallus
Sub-species	G. g. murghi

Distribution

This subspecies found in Northern India and Central Part of the India extending eastward to Orrissa and West Bengal.

Phenotypic Appearance

In its outward aspect, this subspecies is very similar to the previous one: it displays white, slightly smaller earlobes, very sharp neck and saddle hackles of a very deep yellow, the longest of which tend to turn gold and have a rather wide black stripe in the middle. The hen does not differ significantly from the previously described, except for the smaller earlobes.

Burmese red jungle fowl

Taxonomic Classification

Kingdom	Animalia
Phylum	Chordata
Class	Aves
Order	Galliformes
Family	Phasianidae
Genus	Gallus
Species	G. gallus
Sub-species	G. g. spadiceus

Distribution

It is native of South West Yunnan, Burma, Siam, with the exception of North East Laos, the Malacca peninsula and the area North of Sumatra. It is also found in Northeastern part of India.

Phenotypic Appearance

This subspecies does not sensibly vary as far as plumage is concerned. Its lanceolates are in the average shorter than the gallus' and its earlobes are small and red. Apart from this, it displays no differences to the nominal subspecies.

Tonkinese red jungle fowl

Taxonomic Classification

Kingdom	Animalia
Phylum	Chordata
Class	Aves
Order	Galliformes
Family	Phasianidae
Genus	Gallus
Species	G. gallus
Sub-species	G. g. jabouillei

Distribution

It is native of Tonkin, South East Yunnan (China) and Northern Annam (now Vietnam).

Phenotypic Appearance

This subspecies has smaller comb and wattles compared to the other ones; also, earlobes are red and small. The plumage's red is darker, the neck hackles are shorter and less sharp; the saddle is mahogany red, while the hackles are small and dark red; the tail is slightly shorter, the neck - very dark - is tinged with orange.

Javan red jungle fowl
Taxonomic Classification

Kingdom	Animalia
Phylum	Chordata
Class	Aves
Order	Galliformes
Family	Phasianidae
Genus	Gallus
Species	G. gallus
Sub-species	G. g. bankiva

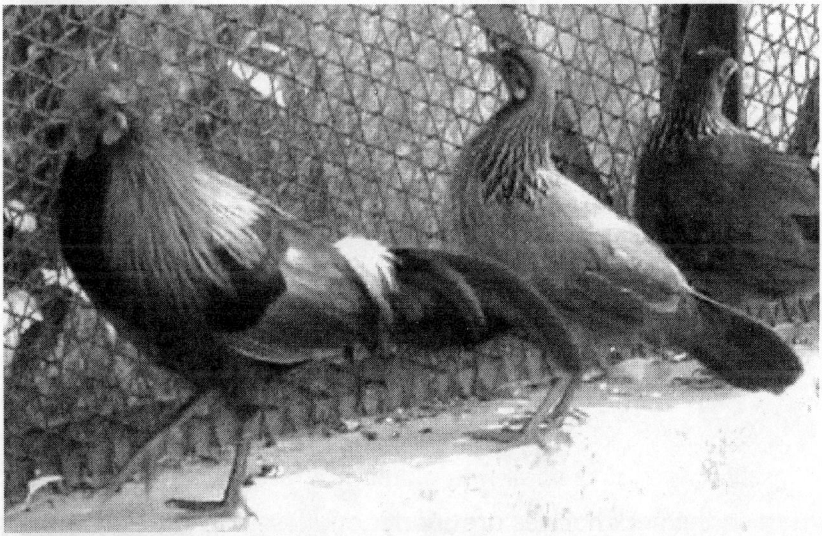

Red Jungle Fowl Male and Female

Distribution

Originally, this subspecies inhabited the South of Sumatra and the islands of Java and Bali. It is likely to have been introduced, however, in the Philippines, Tahiti and as far as Hawaii.

Phenotypic Appearance

Very similar to the Spadiceus subspecies, it is just distinguishable by the neck hackles, that are rather wide and round-edged, a unique characteristic among all subspecies. Earlobes are red with white irregular stripes, the shanks are slate blue.

❑❑❑

Chapter **4**

Origin of Domestic Chicken

There are several views regarding the origin of domestic fowl. Majority believes that the chicken has monophyletic origin and Red junglefowl is its sole ancestor, while some believes that apart from red jungle fowl, other junglefowl(s) might also have contributed towards the origin of domestic chicken, thus it has a polyphyletic origin.

Early evidences for/against the monophyletic origin of chicken

Morphological evidences: Darwin (1896) put the theory of monophyletic origin of chicken on the basis of high similarity between red jungle fowl and some of the early domestic birds, more similarity in voice from RJF and that of domestic fowl; and free and successful mating between RJF and domestic fowl and much better survival of crossbred progenies with good level of fertility on inter-se mating or mating with any of the parents. Further the crossbred offspring had black-red plumage similar to that of *G. gallus*. Spectrogram analysis also show more close resemblance of the crow of the domestic cock with red jungle fowl, while the voice of Grey junglefowl, Green junglefowl or Ceylon junglefowl were quite different.

However, Tegetmeier (1867) felt that Asciatic breeds are quite different from those of Mediterranean origin as they have short wings, a wide dropping tail and are much less flighty. Hence the Asiatic breeds, specially the Cochin had a different origin. Another very major structural difference is the long axis of the occipital foramen (aperture through which the spinal cord emerges from the skull), which is vertical in Cochin breed, while horizontal in Red jungle fowl. The red jungle fowl lacks a silver gene(s), which is dominant type and has sex-linked inheritance in chicken. In many chicken breeds, pair of dominant (S) and recessive (s) alleles of Silver gene exists. While the "S" results in silver plumage, "s" results in gold plumage. Red jungle fowl apparently has only the "s" allele, since silver variants have not been described; whereas the Grey jungle fowl have grey or silver plumage, thus have "S" allele. Further, the production of fertile offspring from the mating of grey jungle fowl and domestic fowl (Ghigi, 1916, 1922) suggested that domestic breeds are not descended from Red junglefowl only. Similar findings were also reported except sterile progenies from Green jungle fowl male and domestic chicken female (Hertwig, 1936).

William Beebe, in his classic "*Monograph of the Pheasants* (1918–1922)" stated that "there can be no doubt that the Red Jungle Fowl alone is the direct ancestor of all our domestic poultry, so this question is removed from the discussion.

Biochemical evidences: Amino acid sequences of well characterized proteins may be a good method to resolve evolutionary relationship between families, orders or classes. Baker et al. (1971), from their extensive studies of egg white proteins through starch gel electrophoresis, concluded that the domestic fowl is derived largely if not entirely from G. gallus. However, consistent difference for glutamyl peptidase between domestic fowl and Red jungle fowl were observed (Baker & Manwell, 1972). Between the Ceylon jungle fowl and Red jungle fowl, differences were observed only in G2 ovoglobulin. Stevens and Duncan (1988) were not convinced with the biochemical evidence on the basis of purity of proteins to homogeneity and the electrophoretic methods.

Complete sequence of the third domain of ovumucoid from domestic fowl, Ceylon junglefowl and Grey jungle fowl were determined and all the three were found to be identical (Laskowski et al. 1987). It generally, requires the sequencing of a large number of different proteins to find the differences between related species and subspecies. This is very time consuming and at present such data are not available.

Domestic fowl was compared with all four junglefowls for four blood group proteins and several other plasma proteins. The genetic distance between the domestic fowl and the four junglefowl species i.e. Red jungle fowl, Grey jungle fowl, Ceylon jungle fowl and Green junglefowl were 0.230, 0.336, 0.658 and 0.681, respectively (Okada et al., 1984), revealing maximum closeness between domestic chicken and red jungle fowl.

Molecular evidences: Early molecular evidences include the presence of indigenous retrovirus RAV-oDNA sequence in red jungle fowl, similar to that in domestic chicken (Weiss and Biggs, 1972), while other species of jungle fowls lack detectable sequences homologous to those of chicken (Frisby et al., 1979).

Based on mtDNA sequences of the D-loop regions from three sub species of red junglefowl i.e. *Gallus gallus gallus, Gallus gallus spadiceus* and *Gallus gallus bankiva; Gallus varius; Gallus lafayettei; Gallus sonneratii;* and domestic breeds (*Gallus gallus domesticus*) evolutionary relationship was established between domestic chicken and four jungle fowl species (Fumihito et al., 1996). At the first glance, *G. varius* appears to be the most divergent of the four species, however it is likely that *G. varius, G. gallus, G. sonneratii*, and *G. lafayettei* branched out from the common stem almost simultaneously in the evolutionary time scale. Split should have occurred shortly thereafter in Gallus of Indian subcontinent to yield a mainland species (*G. sonneratii*) and an island species (*G. lafayettei*).

The restriction endonuclease cleavage patterns of mtDNA were used for evolutionary relationship between four jungle fowls. Sequence divergence between Gallus gallus and G. sonnerati, G. varius and G. lafayattei was 0.9. 10.5 and 12.6 % respectively. Assuming that the rate of evolution of mt DNA is 3 % per million years, It was estimated that the divergence of mtDNA of G. gallus from that of G. sonnerati, G. varius and G. lafayattei occurred 0.3, 3.5 and 4.5 million years ago, respectively.

The phylogenetic analysis of the entire mtDNA genome and nuclear DNA (nucDNA) regions for four CR1 (chicken repeat 1) regions and OTC (ornithine carbamoyl transferase) revealed evidence for hybridization of grey jungle fowl with chickens, red jungle fowl, and La Fayette's jungle fowl. In particular, the analysis of the entire mtDNA genome showed that two grey jungle fowls (GyJF) were clustered in a clade with RJFs and chicken, and that one GyJF was located in a remote position close to Ceylon jungle fowl (CJF). The analyses based on the nuclear sequences revealed that alleles of GyJFs were alternatively clustered with those of CJF and with those of RJFs and chicken. Alternative clustering of RJF and chicken alleles were also observed. These findings taken together strongly indicate that inter-species hybridizations have occurred between GyJF and

RJF/chicken and between GyJF and CJF (Nishibori et al., 2005).

Domestic chickens with yellow skin are homozygous for a recessive allele while, white skinned chickens carry the dominant allele. It was found that yellow skin is caused by regulatory mutation(s) that inhibit expression of the beta-carotene dioxygenase 2 (BCDO2) enzyme in skin, but not in other tissues. A phylogenetic analysis, however, demonstrates that though the white skin allele originates from the red junglefowl, the yellow skin allele originates from a different species, most likely the grey jungle fowl (Errikson et al., 2008). This is the first conclusive evidence for a hybrid origin of the domestic chicken, and it has important implications for our views of the domestication process.

Within Gallus gallus several subspecies namely, from west to east *G. g. murghi*, *G. g. spadiceus*, *G. g. jabouillei*, *G. g. gallus*, *G. g. bankiva*, could have contributed to the domestic stock. However, mitochondrial DNA information obtained in the 1990's suggest that one continental population of red jungle fowl Gallus gallus gallus, probably from Thailand, is likely at the maternal origin of all domestic chicken (Fumihito et al., 1994, 1996).

However, other subspecies of *G. gallus*, *Gallus gallus murghi* and *Gallus gallus jabouillei*, were not included in the present study, the validity of their subspecies status still remain as an open question.

It was found that a 60-bp-long unit containing the nearly invariant tetradecamer, AACTATGAATGGTT, in its center of the D-loop region is duplicated only in members of the genus Gallus and not in other phasianine birds. In the case of *G. varius*, two to four copies were found, while in all *G. lafayettei* as well as *G. sonneratii* birds, three copies were found. All the *G. gallus* birds, regardless of the subspecies, have two copies and also all the domestic fowls had the same copy number as *G. gallus*, again implying that the genealogical origin of the domestic fowls is monophyletic descending from *G. gallus* alone (Fumihito et al., 1994, 1996). Based on 539 bases of mitochondrial DNA D-loop region of six domestic chicken breeds (30 individuals), red jungle fowl, grey jungle fowl, green jungle fowl and Lafayette's jungle fowl, the phylogenetic trees revealed that the red jungle fowl in Thailand and its neighbour areas sufficed as the matriarchic ancestor of Chinese domestic fowls (Fu et al., 2001, Niu et al. 2002).

However, mtDNA work on Japanese gamecocks showed four distinct phylogenetic clades (Komiyama et al., 2003). These results revealed several important new clues about the domestication of chickens suggesting that the monophyletic origin conclusions from early studies might result from incomplete sampling of domestic chickens and red jungle fowl. Mitochondrial DNA hypervariable segment I (HVS-I) sequences from 834 domestic chickens (*Gallus gallus domesticus*) across Eurasia as well as 66 wild red jungle fowls (*Gallus gallus*) from Southeast Asia and China were analysed (Liu et al., 2006). Phylogenetic analyses revealed nine highly divergent mtDNA clades (A–I) in which seven clades contained both the red jungle fowls and domestic chickens. There was no breed-specific clade in the chickens. The clades A, B, and E are distributed ubiquitously in Eurasia, while the other clades were restricted to South and Southeast Asia. Clade C was mainly distributed in Japan and Southeast China, while clades F and G were exclusive to Yunnan, China. The geographic distribution of clade D was closely related to the distribution of the pastime of cock fighting. Statistical tests detect population expansion within each subclade. These distinct distribution patterns and expansion signatures suggest that different clades may originate from different regions, such as Yunnan, South and Southwest China and/or surrounding areas (i.e., Vietnam, Burma, and Thailand), and the Indian subcontinent, respectively, which support the theory of multiple origins in South and Southeast Asia.

In most of the studies, non-inclusion of Indian red jungle fowl (RJF), Gallus gallus murghi has left a big gap in understanding the relationship of this major group of birds. A total of 76 Indian birds that included 56 *G. g. murghi* (RJF), 16 *G. g. domesticus* (domestic chicken) and 4 *G. sonneratii* (Grey JF) were analyzed using both microsatellite markers and mitochondrial D-loop sequences. The D-loop sequences of Indian birds were also compared with those of 779 birds obtained from GenBank. The microsatellite-based phylogenetic trees showed a clear separation of *G. g. domesticus* from *G. g. murghi*, and *G. sonneratii*. Mitochondrial DNA based mismatch distribution analyses showed a lower Harpending's raggedness index in both *G. g. murghi* (0.001515) and in Indian *G. g. domesticus* (0.0149) birds indicating population expansion. When meta analysis of global populations of 855 birds was carried out using median joining haplotype network, 43 Indian birds of G. g. domesticus (19 haplotypes) were distributed throughout the network sharing haplotypes with the RJFs of different origins. These results are suggestive of the occurrence of domestication of chicken independently in different locations of Asia including India. Domestication of chicken from *G. g. spadiceus* and *G. g. gallus* as well as from *G. g. murghi* in India corroborate multiple domestication of Indian and other domestic chicken. In contrast to the commonly held view that RJF and domestic birds hybridize in nature, the present study shows that *G. g. murghi* is relatively pure. Further, the study also suggested that the chicken populations have undergone population expansion, especially in the Indus valley (Kanginakudru et al., 2008).

Phylogenetic analysis based on DNA sequences from 30 introns at 25 nuclear loci from 19 individual samples covering various chicken breeds, red jungle fowl (*G. g. gallus*), and green junglefowl (*G. varius*) shows that the DNA sequences of chickens, red and green junglefowls formed reciprocally monophyletic clusters. The Markov chain Monte Carlo simulation further reveals that domestic chickens diverged from red jungle fowl

58,000±16,000 years ago, well before the archeological dating of domestication, and that their common ancestor in turn diverged from green jungle fowl 3.6 million years ago. Several shared haplotypes nonetheless found between green junglefowl and chickens are attributed to recent unidirectional introgression of chickens into green junglefowl. Shared haplotypes are more frequently found between red junglefowl and chickens, which are attributed to both introgression and ancestral polymorphisms. In conclusion, domestic chickens are closely related to red junglefowl, although genetic contribution from other jungle fowls remains to be answered (Sawai et al., 2010).

❑❑❑

Chapter 5

Molecular Characterization using DNA Markers

It is quite evident that a huge amount of genetic variation exists in all eukaryotic genome. The assaying this genetic variation through some protocol has developed the concept of molecular marker. Hence, a genetic or molecular marker is a site of heterozygosity for some type of neutral DNA variation. Neutral variations are that which are not associated with any measurable phenotypic variation. Such DNA locus or fragments are called genetic/ DNA marker. There are several types of DNA markers and these markers can be classified into two types i.e. Type I and Type II. While Type I markers are associated with a gene of known function, Type II markers seems to have association with anonymous gene segments of one sort or another.

DNA-based markers could alternatively be grouped into clone/sequence based (CSB) markers and fingerprint (FP) markers (Dodgson *et al.*, 1997). The first category requires the isolation of a cloned DNA fragment and often determination of some, if not all of its DNA sequence. The CSB markers include microsatellites, RFLP, STS and EST among others. The FP markers require no prior knowledge of the sequence of the polymorphic region or isolation of a cloned DNA fragment and they include RAPD, VNTRs, AFLP, RLGS and many others. The FP markers are inherently Type II markers, whereas, CSB markers include both Type I and Type II markers. Of the CSB markers, microsatellite markers are predominant markers and are more commonly used for genome mapping, detection of polymorphism among individuals, estimation of genetic similarity/ relatedness among and within populations.

Further, markers may be random or specific. The markers which detect the sequence variability at one or more loci, but do not able to give the location of this variability are random markers. The VNTRs and RAPD are the good example of random markers. The specific markers, detects the sequence variability in a known region e.g. Microsatellite or Simple Sequence Repeat (SSR) markers.

Genetic polymorphism between RJF and domestic chicken using different markers

Two males and 3 females of Red Jungle Fowl (RJF) and 5 males and 5 females from each of six chicken breeds namely White Leghorn (WL), Rhodes Island Red (RIR), White Plymouth Rock (WR), Red Cornish (RC), Aseel (AS) and Kadaknath (KN) were included. Total of 20 arbitrary short oligonucleotide primers (10 mer) with GC content of 60-70%, 3 MASA primers (16-18 bp) having minisatellite consensus sequences viz. OAT 18.2, 0 33.15 and microsatellite sequence viz. $(GTG)_5$ and 8 microsatellite markers were used (Tomar et al., 2007).

Out of 20 random primers used, 18 detected polymorphism between the RJF and other chicken breeds. Out of 119 bands amplified, 57 bands (~ 48 %) were polymorphic. The average number of total bands amplified per primer was 4.90, 4.95, 5.10, 4.85, 5.10, 5.05, 5.35 in RJF, WL, RIR, RC, WR, AS, KN, respectively. The proportion of the primers capable of detecting the polymorphism among the populations depends upon the genetic background of the populations, genetic distances between the populations and complexity of the genome. Very high percentage of polymorphic primers in present study might be due to use of selective RAPD primers, however when the RAPD primers are selected randomly, comparatively lower proportion of primers were found to be polymorphic. The amplification profiles showed the resolution of 3-10 bands in the size range of 400 to 4000 bp.

A total of 3 oligonucleotide primers (15-32 mer) commonly used for classical DNA fingerprinting experiments viz. O33.15 (minisatellite); OAT 18.2 and $(GTG)_5$ (micro-satellite) DNA sequences were used as a single primer. The total numbers of bands amplified were 11, 13, and 7 with O33.15, OAT 18.2 and $(GTG)_5$, respectively. These band ranged in the size range of 395 to 2523 bp. Proportion of polymorphic loci was 73 %, 23 % and 14 % with primer O33.15, OAT 18.2 and GTG_5, respectively. Overall a total of 31 loci amplified and 12 of these (39%) were found to be polymorphic. The average numbers of total bands amplified per primer were 8.00, 8.00, 9.33, 8.66, 9.33, 9.66 and 9.00 in RJF, WL, RIR, RC, WR, AS and KN, respectively. These bands ranged in the size range of from 395 to 2523 bp in RJF, 395 to 2116 bp in WL, 395 to 2523 bp in RIR, 395 to 2264 bp in RC, 395 to 2523 bp in WR, 395 to 2523 bp in AS and 395 to 2523 bp in KN.

Out of 8 microsatellite markers, only five markers generated distinct amplification. A total of 25 alleles were amplified from the 5 micro satellite markers, giving an average of 5 alleles per locus. The number of alleles per locus amplified ranged from 3 (LEI 113) to 6 alleles (ADL 237 and LEI 65). The difference in allele size varied from 18 bp (in loci LEI113 and ROS54) to 88 bp (in locus ADL 237). In general, the size of alleles ranged from 96 bp to 290 bp and the majority of alleles were in the size range of 110 bp to 2756 bp. All the 5 markers were polymorphic, however no species specific allele could be identified. Hence, the microsatellite markers seemed to be more informative and appropriate for genetic polymorphism studies populations.

Microsatellite allelic profile of Indian RJF

A total of 25 polymorphic microsatellite markers (15 tetra-nucleotides and 10 di-nucleotides) were used to develop allelic profile of Indian Red junglefowl (RJF) and domestic chicken represented by three breeds i.e. White Leghorn (WLH) as egg-type, Aseel (AS) as game-type and Red Cornish (RC) as meat-type (Vinay, 2010). A total of 475 alleles with an average of 19 alleles per locus were produced with 25 microsatellite markers. The highest numbers of 248 alleles with an average of 9.92 alleles per locus were observed in RJF followed by 212 alleles with an average of 8.48 alleles per locus in AS, 177 alleles with an average of 7.08 alleles per locus in each of WLH and RC populations. The number of alleles at each locus ranged from 5 (MCW111) to 43 (LEI 212). The RJF population showed higher values of means of expected heterozygosity (HE), observed heterozygosity (Ho) and Polymorphic Information Content (PIC) i.e. 0.7975, 0.4565, 0.7716, respectively as compared to the three domestic chicken populations.

Population specific alleles

A total of 242 population specific alleles with allelic frequency ranged from 0.0250 to

0.8333 were detected across the RJF and three domestic chicken breeds with all 25 microsatellite loci. Out of these 242 population specific alleles, 103 were specific to RJF, 44 were specific to WLH, 56 were specific to AS and 39 were specific to RC. Out of 242 population specific alleles, majority of the alleles (~75 %) were present in low to very low frequency and only 61 alleles were found in a frequency of more than 0.10. Among these 61 alleles, we found 29 population specific alleles in the range of allelic frequency 0.100 to 0.500 in RJF, 12 in RC (0.111 to 0.647), 10 in WLH (0.100 to 0.575) and also 10 in RC (0.100 to 0.833). Among the 29 RJF specific alleles, only 4 alleles, i.e. ADL120-178bp, ADL265-114bp, MCW111-104 and MCW111-106 bp seemed to have some practical importance as these alleles are present in very good allelic frequency range of 0.500 to 0.526. In domestic chicken breeds, three alleles i.e. LEI243-186 in WLH, LEI214-140 in AS and LEI229-193 in RC were more important from the breed identification point of view. Considering all the chicken population together, there are 226 alleles, which are present in domesticated chicken, but absent in RJF.

ADL 120

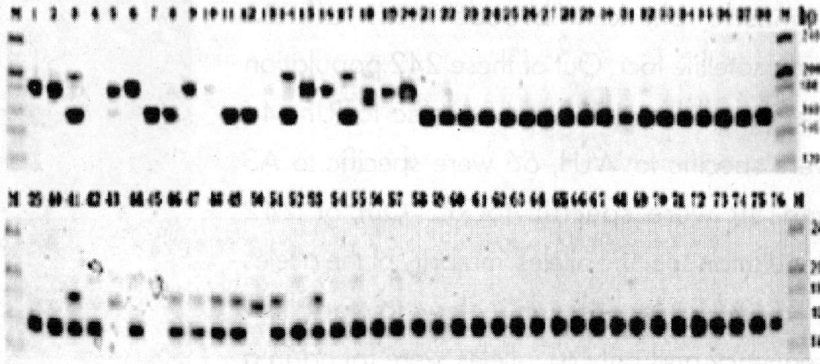

LEI 217

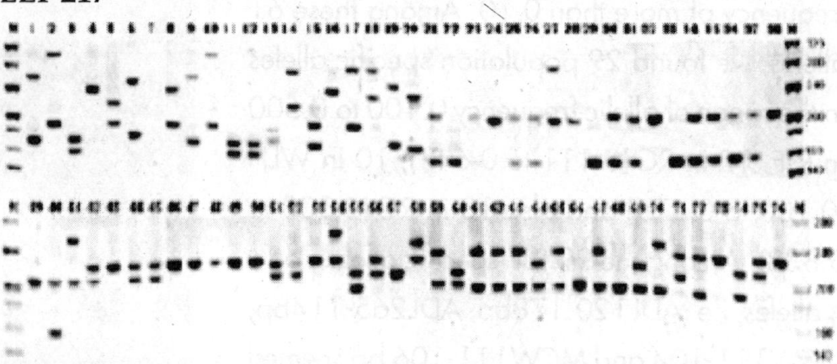

LEI 229

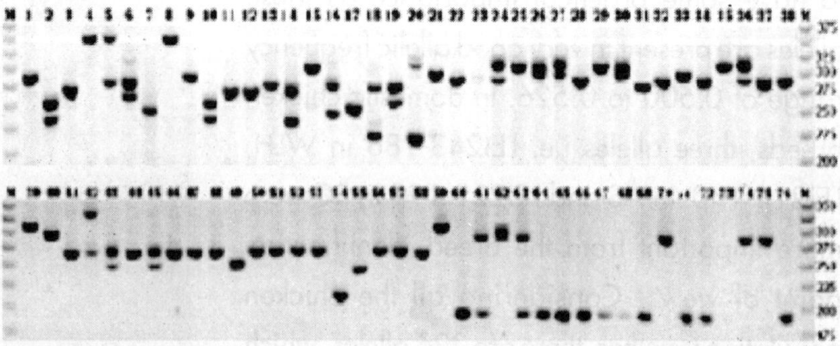

Fig. 5.1 : Microsatellite allelic profile of Indian RJF and different Chicken populations. Lane 1-20 : Red Jungle Fowl, 21-40 : White Leghorn, 41-58 : Aseel, 59-76 : Red Cornish. M : 20 bp DNA ladder

Table 5.1 : Population-specific alleles in RJF, White Leghorn (WLH), Aseel (AS) and Red Cornish (RC) at various microsatellite loci

Locus	Population specific alleles			
	RJF	WLH	Aseel	RC
ADL34	-	125(0.0526) 151(0.0263)	149(0.1667) 159(0.0278)	113(0.0882) 153(0.0294)
ADL120	178(0.5000) 182(0.1053) 192(0.0789)	-	146(0.0882) 148(0.0882) 150(0.4118) 168(0.0588) 170(0.0558) 172(0.1471) 174(0.0558)	-
ADL158	172(0.0263) 174(0.0263) 176(0.0789)	-	-	208(0.1471)
ADL209	160(0.0714)	-	138(0.0333) 140(0.1000)	132(0.0417) 158(0.0417) 166(0.0417) 178(0.0417)
ADL254	-	-	152(0.0278) 156(0.0278) 166(0.0278) 168(0.0556) 170(0.0833) 172(0.0278) 176(0.0278) 180(0.0278)	162(0.0294)
ADL265	108(0.0263) 114(0.5263) 128(0.0263)	130(0.1500) 136(0.0250) 144(0.0250)	100(0.1944)	-
ADL270	90(0.1053) 106(0.0526)	-	116(0.1176) 126(0.0588)	130(0.0313) 132(0.0625)
ADL327	126(0.0526)	-	102(0.0278) 122(0.1111) 130(0.0278)	100(0.0294) 110(0.3529) 120(0.0294)

				124(0.0294) 98(0.0882)
ADL331	161(0.1471)	169(0.0250)	173(0.0278) 183(0.0556)	181(0.1111) 195(0.0278)
LEI194	118(0.0500) 138(0.0500) 182(0.1250) 184(0.2250)	150(0.0250) 156(0.0250) 168(0.0250)	144(0.0294) 166(0.0882)	-
LEI209	136(0.0250) 162(0.0250)	142(0.0750)	184(0.0278) 188(0.0556) 192(0.0278) 196(0.0278)	-
LEI212	294(0.0263) 362(0.0263) 372(0.0263) 376(0.0526) 378(0.0263) 382(0.0789) 384(0.0526) 394(0.0263) 396(0.0526) 402(0.0263) 404(0.0263) 406(0.0263) 408(0.0789) 414(0.1316) 424(0.0526) 434(0.0263) 440(0.0789) 444(0.0263)	336(0.1471) 342(0.0294) 432(0.0588) 452(0.20590 456(0.0294) 484(0.0294)	322(0.0278) 370(0.1944) 386(0.0556) 422(0.0278) 458(0.0556) 492(0.0278)	388(0.0278) 412(0.3333)
LEI214	148(0.3421) 172(0.0263) 184(0.0263) 186(0.0263) 188(0.0263) 192(0.0526) 196(0.0526) 200(0.0526) 204(0.1842) 208(0.0526) 224(0.0263)	-	140(0.8333)	134(0.0588) 156(0.3529) 288(0.1471) 308(0.0882) 312(0.0882) 332(0.0588)

LEI217	158(0.0263) 160(0.0263) 164(0.1053) 168(0.0526) 172(0.0526) 176(0.0263) 180(0.0263) 188(0.1579) 260(0.0263) 268(0.0789) 300(0.0526)	148(0.3750) 272(0.0250)	252(0.0278) 264(0.0278)	192(0.0556)
LEI221	120(0.0263) 160(0.0526) 164(0.0263) 204(0.0526) 208(0.0263) 216(0.0263) 220(0.0263)	232(0.0526) 236(0.0278) 240(0.0278) 244(0.0278)	212(0.0588)	-
LEI228	190(0.0250) 254(0.0250) 266(0.0250)	198(0.0250) 238(0.1000)	222(0.0294)	-
LEI229	220(0.0750) 238(0.0750) 256(0.0750) 274(0.2500) 355(0.1250)	-	211(0.0526)	193(0.6471)
LEI232	184(0.0278) 206(0.0556) 228(0.0556) 232(0.0278)	202(0.0556) 276(0.0556) 280(0.0278) 284(0.0278) 290(0.0278)	-	178(0.0833)
LEI234	232(0.3000) 264(0.1250) 268(0.2000) 272(0.1500)	296(0.0750)	216(0.0833)	260(0.0556) 276(0.2500) 328(0.0278) 364(0.0556) 388(0.0556)
LEI237	283(0.0526) 287(0.1053) 303(0.0789) 335(0.0789)	211(0.1053) 215(0.2105) 219(0.0263) 291(0.0526)	279(0.1111)	-

		363(0.0526) 383(0.0268) 387(0.0789) 391(0.0526)		
LEI243	172(0.0750) 182(0.0250) 190(0.0500) 208(0.1000) 316(0.0500) 320(0.1000) 328(0.0500) 332(0.0250)	186(0.5750)	170(0.0278)	176(0.0278) 308(0.2222) 312(0.2222) 364(0.0278)
LEI246	243(0.1316)	247(0.0526) 263(0.0263) 267(0.0526) 271(0.1053)	-	199(0.1667)
LEI248			222(0.0278) 258(0.0833) 262(0.0556)	
LEI192	274(0.2778) 370(0.2222) 393(0.1111) 401(0.1667) 465(0.1111)	270(0.1500)	283(0.0556) 286(0.0833) 287(0.0556) 332(0.0278) 417(0.0556)	347(0.1667)
MCW111	104(0.5000) 106(0.5000)	-	-	-
Total	103	44	56	39

Allelic profile of Indian RJF with AFLP markers

The AFLP assay was performed using *Taq*I restriction endonuclease enzyme. The sequences of *Eco*RI and *Taq*I adapters and primers used in the AFLP assay described here are shown in table 5.2. To produce *Eco*RI/*Taq*I AFLP marker, each 400 ng genomic DNA sample was digested using *Eco*RI and *Taq*I restriction enzymes followed by adapter ligation. This was served as template for the pre-amplification reaction. For pre-amplification reaction 5µl of template DNA was then added to a pre-amplification mix containing all PCR components with 15 pmol each of *Eco*RI primer +A and *Taq*I primer +A carrying one selective nucleotide, in a total of 50 µl. These diluted reaction products serve as templates for the final selective amplification reactions using primers with three/four selective bases in one or both primers (Vinay, 2010).

Table 5.2 : Sequences of adapters & primers used in AFLP analysis

Specifications	Name	5'-3' sequences
Adaptors		
Eco*RI adaptors*	Top strand	5'-CTCGTAGACTGCGTACC
	Bottom strand	5'-AATTGGTACGCAGTCTAC
*Taq*I adapters	Top strand	5'-GACGATGAGTCCTGAC
	Bottom strand	5'-CGGTCAGGACTCAT
Primers		
*Eco*RI primer		5'-GACTGCGTACCAATTC
*Taq*I primer		5'-GATGAGTCCTGACCGA
Pre-amplification primers		
*Eco*RI primer +A		5'-GACTGCGTACCAATTCA
*Taq*I primer +A		5'-GATGAGTCCTGACCGAA

***Eco*RI Selective amplification primers**		
*Eco*RI primer +ATA	E01	5′-GACTGCGTACCAATTCATA
*Eco*RI primer +AGC	E02	5′-GACTGCGTACCAATTCAGC
*Eco*RI primer +ACA	E03	5′-GACTGCGTACCAATTCACA
*Eco*RI primer +AGT	E04	5′-GACTGCGTACCAATTCAGT
***Taq*I Selective amplification primers**		
*Taq*I primer +AAT	T01	5′-GATGAGTCCTGACCGAAAT
*Taq*I primer +ACT	T02	5′-GATGAGTCCTGACCGAACT
*Taq*I primer +AAG	T03	5′-GATGAGTCCTGACCGAAAG
*Taq*I primer +AGC	T04	5′-GATGAGTCCTGACCGAAGC
*Taq*I primer +ATG	T05	5′-GATGAGTCCTGACCGAATG
*Taq*I primer +ATGT	T06	5′-GATGAGTCCTGACCGAATGT

The final products were resolved on 3.5% metaphor (Lonza, Rockland, ME USA) gel in 1X TBE buffer. The gels were stained with ethidium bromide and scanned and photographed by a Phosphor-imager (FLA-5100, Fluorescent/ Radioisotope Science Imaging System, Fugifilm, Japan). Molecular sizes of AFLP markers were estimated by using 20 bp DNA ladder (Bangalore Genei) as external molecular size marker.

A total of 20 primer combinations using four *Eco*RI selective primers and six *Taq*I selective combinations were used. A total of 318 scorable AFLP bands in the range of 50-500 bps were detected across the populations. Out of which, 309 (97.17%) were polymorphic bands. In RJF population, a total of 311 bands could be scored. Out of which, 302 (97%) were found polymorphic. In WLH population, a total of 270 bands could be scored. Out of which, 60 (22%) were found polymorphic. In AS population, a total of 282 bands could be scored. Out of which, 105 (37%) were found polymorphic. In RC population, a total of 281 bands could be scored. Out of which, 57 (20%) were found polymorphic.

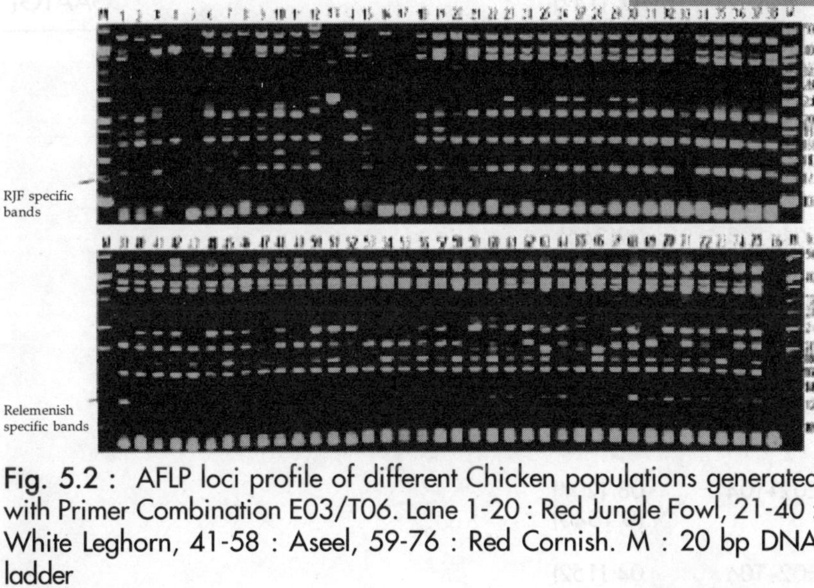

Fig. 5.2 : AFLP loci profile of different Chicken populations generated with Primer Combination E03/T06. Lane 1-20 : Red Jungle Fowl, 21-40 : White Leghorn, 41-58 : Aseel, 59-76 : Red Cornish. M : 20 bp DNA ladder

Population specific alleles

A total of 29 population specific AFLP bands were observed in all 4 populations using 20 *Eco*RI/*Taq*I primer combinations. In RJF, 13 out of 20 Primer combinations generated 26

Table 5.3 : Population-specific AFLP markers in Red jungle Fowl (RJF), White Leghorn (WL), Aseel (AS) and Red Cornish (RC) with various AFLP primer combinations.

Primer Combination	Population-specific AFLP fragments (fragment number with their respective sizes (in bps) and allele frequencies per population			
	RJF	WLH	AS	RC
E01+T02	01(057) (0.0253)			
	02 (061) (0.0780)			
	09 (149) (0.2254)			
	10 (162) (0.1056)			
	17 (260) (0.0513)			
E01+T03	09(265) (0.3292)			
E02+T02	03 (108) (0.0780)			
E02+T03			08 (142) (0.4226)	
E02+T04	08 (204) (0.1340)			
E02+T06	04 (152) (0.1340)			
	08 (277) (0.0513)			
E03+T02	10 (311) (0.0513)			05 (230) (0.1181)
E03+T03	03 (126) (0.2745)			

	09 (218) (0.0823)			
E03+T04	03 (082) (0.0780)			
	09 (147) (0.1398)			
E03+T05	01 (079) (0.1340)			
	04 (116) (0.0513)			
	07 (146) (0.1340)			
	13 (223) (0.0513)			
	14 (233) (0.0780)			
E03+T06	04 (146) (0.1340)			
	09 (229) (0.0513)			11 (262) (0.1502)
E04+T02	05 (190) (0.2584)			
	06 (213) (0.0780)			
E04+T05	04 (104) (0.0541)			
Total	26	0	1	2

population specific bands and the number of population specific bands from these primer combinations was ranged from 1-5. In domestic chicken breeds very low number of population bands could be detected. 2 bands in RC and one band in AS were observed. While in WLH population no band was observed as population specific. The 14 out of 29 bands were present in less than 10 % allele frequency, all these bands were found in RJF only. In RJF, E01+T03 –09 AFLP band was found more important from the RJF identification point of view, as this band was present with allele frequency 0.3292. Another important band was found in AS, E02+T03 –08 with allele frequency 0.4226.

□□□

Chapter 6

Mitochondrial DNA Polymorphism

Mitochondrial genome (mtDNA) in vertebrates is a comprised of about 37 genes coding for 22 transfer RNAs (tRNAs), 2 ribosomal RNAs (rRNAs), 13 messenger RNAs (mRNAs) alongwith a non-coding control region, however the gene order within the mtDNA varied among taxa (Desjardins and Morais 1990; Saccone et al. 2000). Within the mitochondrial genome, the control region showed the maximum nucleotide substitution rate as it lacks coding constraints. Hence this region has widely been used for diversity studies.

Sequence and structure of D loop

Complete D loop region was amplified, cloned and sequenced in Indian Red Jungle Fowl

(Ahmed, 2009). The sequencing results revealed tRNA-Glu at 3′ end of, complete 1232 nucleotide of D loop region and tRNA-Phe at 5′ end (Figure 6.1). This gene order in the flanking region of D loop is very well conserved within the genera *Gallus* as well as other Avian order (Desjardins and Moris, 1990; Desjardins et al. 1990 and Quinn and Wilson, 1993) and is different from that observed in mammals, where tRNA Pro is present at 5″ end of D loop (Saccone et al. 1991; Douzery and Randi, 1997).

A plot of number of variable sites in non-overlapping 50 bp segments (Figure 6.2) showed three distinct regions or domains i.e. highly variable domain I (1– 450 nt), highly conserved domain II (451-900 nt) and domain III (901-1298). Presence of three distinct domains, based on the nucleotide variability in the D loop region of Indian RJF is consistent with the presence of three distinct domains in D loop region of Finches (Marshal and Baker, 1997), in *Alectoris* (Randi and Lucchini, 1998) and in vultures (Roqυes et al. 2004). While the domain I showed higher proportion of A+T than G+C, domain II was CT rich (62.4 %) and domain III showed very low proportion of G i.e. 4.7 % and high A+T proportion i.e. 78.4 %. This type of base composition has been shown by most of the avian species (Roques et al. 2004).

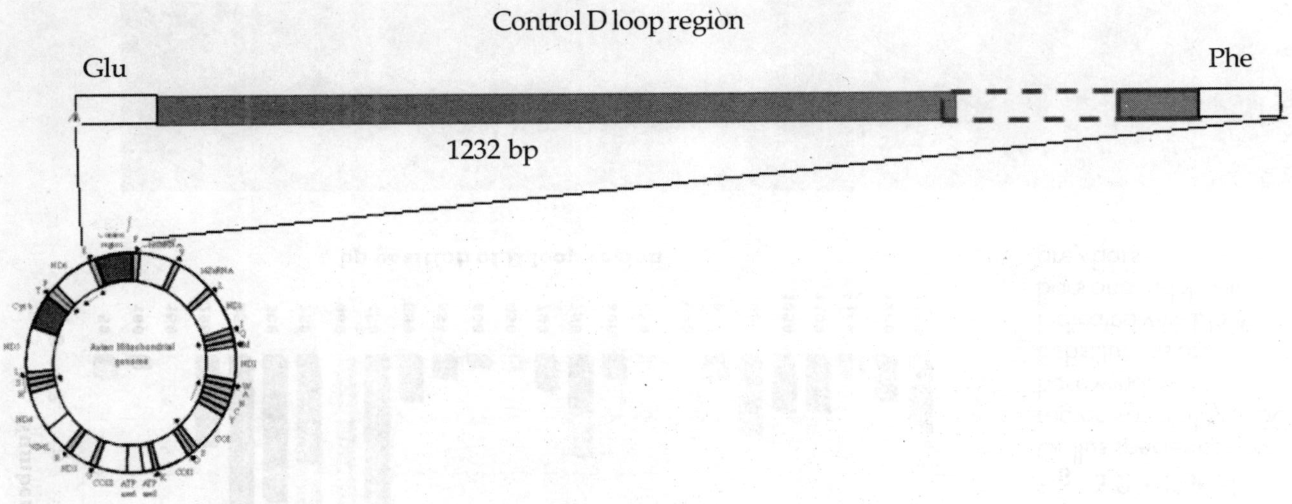

Fig. 6.1 : Diagrammatic representation of Avian mitochondrial DNA and D loop region

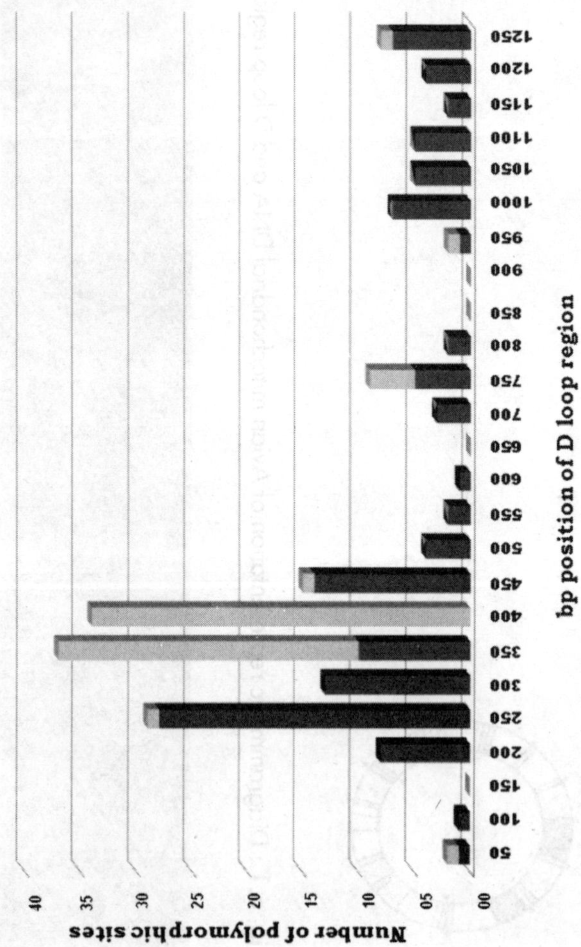

Fig. 6.2 : Plot of Gallus species control region variability in 50 base windows. Substitutions are indicated with black bars and indels with grey bars

Structure and Conserved Sequence Motifs

The sequence alignment of complete D loop region in Indian RJF with other jungle fowls and domestic chicken revealed conservation of different motifs of functional importance Figure 6.3). A sequence capable to form a hairpin structure was identified in first block of domain I and was completely conserved in galliformes. Secondary structure of this hairpin is determined by a stem of seven complementary Cs/Gs and a loop containing a TCCC motif. The TCCC motil was also present in mammalian D loop (Douzery and Randi, 1997) and was associated with termination of H strands (Dufresne et al. 1996). There are two more copies of TCCC, mapping at nt 23-26 and 244-247, which flanked the cloverleaf putative secondary structure formed by single strand domain I. At the 5′ end of the domain I, an interrupted poly-C sequence was observed in the all the Gallus sequences including *G. g. murghi*. This structure seems to be a conserved feature across many species and was described in birds including Struthioniformes, Galliformes, Falconiformes, and Sphenisciformes. The perfectly conserved second block of domain I in Gallus species showed the sequences similar to mammalian TASs. Sbisa et al. (1997) identified two long conserved blocks in domain I of mammalian D loop region i.e. ETAS1 and ETAS2, potentially involved in the control of H strand synthesis. Interestingly, in Gallus genus, a sequence similar to ETAS1 was identified in second block of domain I, but ETAS2 sequence could not be found without ambiguity. Putative TAS sequence has also been identified in domain I of other avian species such as chaffinches and greenfinch (Marshall and Baker, 1997), *Alectoris* ((Randi and Lucchini, 1998) and *G. barbatus* and *N. percnopterus* (Roques et al. 2004).

In domain I, repeats of the tandem sequences, which resembles with CSB1 were identified. Interestingly, these repeats showed variation in repeatability between the *Gallus* species. While all the *G. gallus* sub species as well as *G. varius* showed two repeats, the *G. sonneratti* and *G. lefeyettei* had three repeats. The additional repeat of the tandem sequence increased the size of D loop region in *G. sonneratti* and *G. lefeyettei* to 1288 bp and 1292 bp, respectively against 1227 bp to 1232 bp in other *Gallus* species. Roques et al. (2004) showed that the difference in number of tandem repeats resulted in the differences in the size of D loop region in *N. percnopterus* (2031 bp) and in *G. barbatus* (1750 bp). The single stranded domain I can form potential secondary cloverleaf structures and this structure is highly conserved between Gallus species. The potential secondary cloverleaf structures formed by single-stranded domain I is also well conserved (Desjardins and Morais, 1991; Quinn and Wilson, 1993; Ramirez *et al.*, 1993; Randi and Lucchini, 1998).

The domain II showed very high degree of conserved sequences in the genus *Gallus* and showed the presence of the perfectly conserved F, E, D and C boxes among the *Gallus* genus. These conserved blocks were also reported in other avian species like goose (Quinn and Wilson, 1993), finches (Marshall and Baker, 1997), *Alectoris* (Randi and Lucchini, 1998) and vultures (Roques et al. 2004) as well as in mammals (Sbisa et al. 1997). The domain III also showed several conserved functional sequences in the genus *Gallus*. A poly (C) sequence similar to the O_H of mammals was identified just a few nucleotide downstream from the poutative CSB-I. The CSB-I was absolutely conserved between Gallus species,, however the CSB-II and CSB-III sequences could not be unambiguously identified. Randi and Lucchini (1998) also reported this poly C stretch sequence similar to the OH of mammals in *Alectoris*. The conserved CSB1 block has been identified in the domain III, but CSB2 and CSB 3 could not be identified in this region of other avian species also (Randi and Lucchini, 1998, Marshall and Baker, 1997). The bi-directional LSP/HSP promoters, as identified by L'Abbe et al. (1991) were perfectly conserved in the genus *Gallus*. This sequence contains an almost perfect inverted repeat, which can be folded into stable hairpin. Farther upstream, is the most variable part of the CSB domain, which is rich in poly(T) and poly(A) strings. The LSP/HSP sequences were also identified in Alectoris and were well conserved (Randi and Lucchini (1998).

Allele specific PCR for genotyping the SNP in mitochondrial genome in red jungle fowl and domestic chicken

Single nucleotide polymorphism (SNP), a new type of molecular marker and its more recent concept has basically arisen from the recent need for the densities of genetic markers for the studies of multifactorial diseases and the recent progress in polymorphism detection and genotyping techniques (Ahmed, 2009). Detection of SNPs in the genome is important

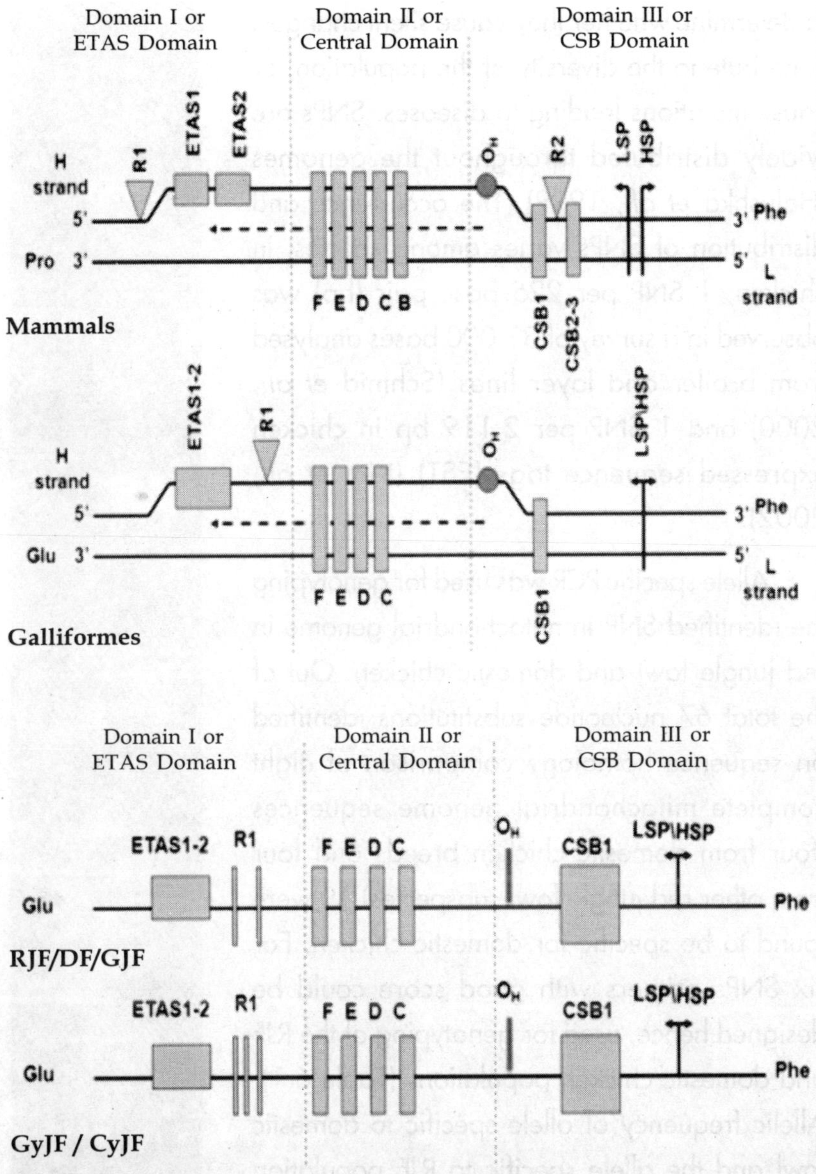

Fig. 6.3 : Comparison of different motips of function importance in different domains between mammals and Galliformes (I) and between different junglefowls including domestic chicken

to determine whether they cause silent changes, contribute to the diversity of the population, or cause mutations leading to diseases. SNPs are widely distributed throughout the genomes (Halushka *et al.*, 1999). The occurrence and distribution of SNPs varies among species. In chicken, 1 SNP per 225 base pair (bp) was observed in a survey of 31,000 bases analysed from broiler and layer lines (Schmid *et al.*, 2000) and 1 SNP per 2,119 bp in chicken expressed sequence tags (EST) (Kim *et al.*, 2002).

Allele specific PCR was used for genotyping the identified SNP in mitochondrial genome in red jungle fowl and domestic chicken. Out of the total 67 nucleotide substitutions identified on sequence homology comparison of eight complete mitochondrial genome sequences (four from domestic chicken breeds and four from other red jungle fowl subspecies) 19 were found to be specific for domestic chicken. For six SNPs primers with good score could be designed hence, used for genotyping of the RJF and domestic chicken populations (Table 6.1). Allelic frequency of allele specific to domestic fowl and the allele specific to RJF population were 0.94 and 0.89 at COI-114-C/T snp; 0.83 and 0.89 at COI-255-G/A snp; 0.78 and 0.94

at COII-279-C/T snp; 0.94 and 0.83 at ATP6-294-G/A SNP; 0.83 and 0.94 at ND4-969-C/T SNP; and 0.94 and 0.78 at CYTB-543-T/C SNP, respectively (Table 6.2). Though the frequency of specific alleles in respective populations was very high, but these alleles were not fixed in the populations hence these SNPs could not be used as population specific markers.

Table 6.1 : Details of the primers used for SNP genotyping

SNP/ Type of PCR	Primer Type	Primer Code	Primer Sequence
COI-114-C/T			
General PCR	Forward	COI-F	ggcttcgatcccatacaattt
	Reverse	COI-R	cggctaaagggggtaaactgt
Allele Specific PCR	Forward	COI-F	ggcttcgatcccatacaattt
	Reverse	COI-114-R-RJF	ggctgtcctagttctgcgcgg
	Reverse	COI-114-R-RJF	ggctgtcctagttctgcgcga
COI-255-G/A			
General PCR	Forward	COI-F	ggcttcgatcccatacaattt
	Reverse	COI-R	cggctaaagggggtaaactgt
Allele Specific PCR	Forward	COI-F	ggcttcgatcccatacaattt
	Reverse	COI-255-R-RJF	tctggggcaccgattataagc
	Reverse	COI-255-R-RJF	tctggggcaccgattataagt
COII-279-C/T			
General PCR	Forward	COII-F	ggccaaccactcccaactag
	Reverse	COII-R	agggattgcgtctgtttttacc
Allele Specific PCR	Forward	COII-279-F-RJF	agacgaaatcgacgaacctgat
	Forward	COII-279-F-DF	agacgaaatcgacgaacctgac
	Reverse	COII-R	agggattgcgtctgtttttacc

ATP6-294-G/A			
General PCR	Forward	ATP6-F	atccctctaatcctcccatcact
	Reverse	ATP6-R	gggcgattgtggctgtagaga
Allele Specific PCR	Forward	ATP6-294-F-RJF	ccttcaccccaactacccaact
	Forward	ATP6-294-F-DF	ccttcaccccaactacccagct
	Reverse	ATP6-R	gggcgattgtggctgtagaga
ND4-969-C/T			
General PCR	Forward	ND4-F	gcccatgtagaagcaccaatc
	Reverse	ND4-R	gtgggggaggatcagttgaagag
Allele Specific PCR	Forward	ND4-F	gcccatgtagaagcaccaatc
	Reverse	ND4-969-R-RJF	gctaggcagaataaagggaaga
	Reverse	ND4-969-R-DF	gctaggcagaataaagggagga
CYTB-543-T/C			
General PCR	Forward	CYTB-F	cccacacttgccggaacgtac
	Reverse	CYTB-R	ggggtgagtatgagagttaagcc
Allele Specific PCR	Forward	CYTB-F	cccacacttgccggaacgtac
	Reverse	CYTB-543-R-RJF	caaaggggaggaggaagtgtaag
	Reverse	CYTB-543-R-DF	caaaggggaggaggaagtgtaaa

Table 6.2 : Allelic frequency at different SNP positions in RJF and domestic fowl

SNP	Population	Presumed allele	Allelic frequency
COI-114-C/T	Domestic Fowl	C	0.94
	Red Jungle Fowl	T	0.89
COI-255-G/A	Domestic Fowl	G	0.83
	Red Jungle Fowl	A	0.89
COII-279-C/T	Domestic Fowl	C	0.78
	Red Jungle Fowl	T	0.94
ATP6-294-G/A	Domestic Fowl	G	0.89
	Red Jungle Fowl	A	0.83
ND4-969-C/T	Domestic Fowl	C	0.83
	Red Jungle Fowl	T	0.94
CYTB-543-T/C	Domestic Fowl	T	0.94
	Red Jungle Fowl	C	0.78

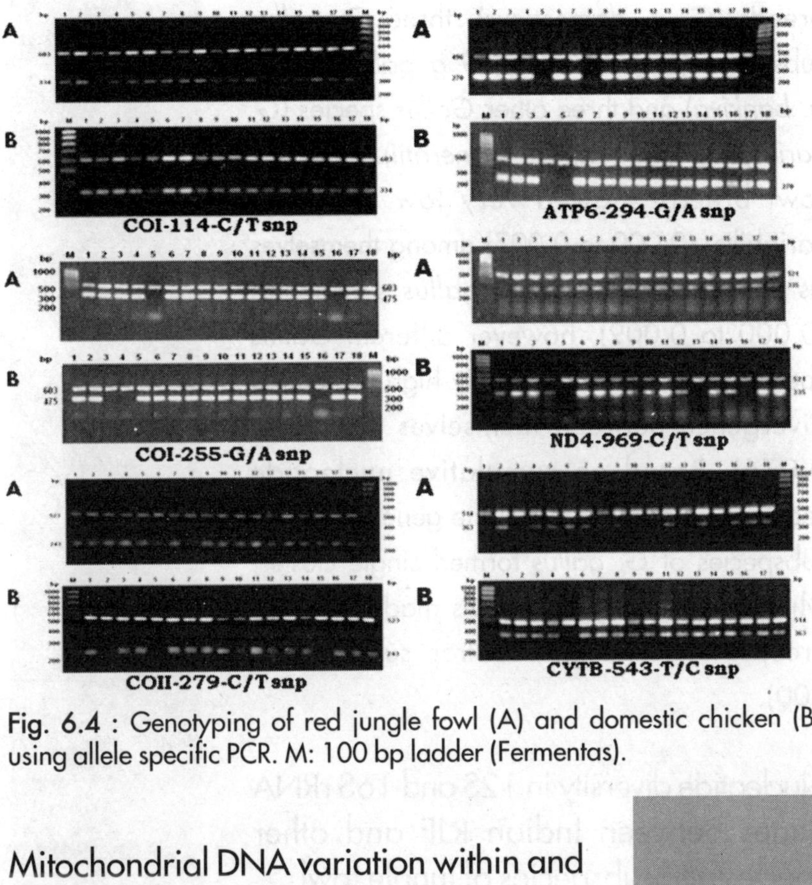

Fig. 6.4 : Genotyping of red jungle fowl (A) and domestic chicken (B) using allele specific PCR. M: 100 bp ladder (Fermentas).

Mitochondrial DNA variation within and between the Gallus species

Nucleotide sequence variation in two ribosomal genes (12S rRNA and 16S rRNA), two ATPase genes (ATPase 6 and ATPase 8), three Cytochrome Oxidase genes (COI, COII & COIII), one Cytochrome B gene (Cytb) and 7 NADP dehrdrogenase genes (ND1, ND2, ND3, ND4, ND4L, ND5 and ND6) was used to estimate genetic diversity between domestic fowl breeds (*G. g. domesticus*), three *G. gallus* subspecies (*G. g. spadicus, G. g. gallus* and *G. g. bankiva*) and three other *Gallus* species (*G. varius, G. lafayetei, G. sonneratii*). Domestic fowl breeds showed very low sequence variability (0.000 to 0.007) among themselves as well as with other *G. gallus* subspecies (0.000 to 0.009), however different *Gallus* species showed comparatively high nucleotide divergence between themselves (0.016 to 0.076). Based on cumulative nucleotide sequence variability for all the genes, different subspecies of *G. gallus* formed single cluster, while other three jungle fowls made separate group with very high bootstrap support (71-100).

Nucleotide diversity in 12S and 16S rRNA genes between Indian RJF and other species and subspecies of jungle fowl

Nucleotide sequence variation in two ribosomal genes (12S rRNA and 16S rRNA) used to estimate genetic diversity between Indian Red Jungle Fowl (G. gallus murghi), *G. gallus* subspecies (*G. g. spadicus, G. g. gallus* and *G. g. bankiva*) including *G. g. domesticus* (domestic fowl) and three other *Gallus* species (*G. varius, G. lafayetei, G. sonneratii*). The

Jukes-Cantor genetic distance estimates between *G. g. murghi* and the domestic fowl breeds as well as other *G. gallus* subspecies were very low and ranged from 0.005 to 0.007, while the genetic distances between *G. g. murghi* and other three jungle fowls were high (0.035 to 0.042). Similarly, for 16 S RNA, very low nucleotide sequence variation was observed between the *G. g. murghi* and other *G. gallus* subspecies including *G. g. domesticus* (genetic distances = 0.000 to 0.003). However, *G. g. murghi* showed higher genetic distances with other three jungle fowls (0.015 to 0.029). The NJ phylogenetic tree showed the *G. g. murghi* with domestic fowl breeds and other *G. gallus* subspecies in one cluster with a good bootstrap support (> 60 %), while other jungle fowls made separate groups.

❏❏❏

Chapter 7

Cytokines

Cytokines are proteins or peptides secreted by the cells that play a key role in immune and inflammatory responses through activation and regulation of other cells and tissues. Until recently, only a limited number of immune regulator and effector genes and their encoded polypeptides were identified in avian species due to the low level of sequence homologies with their mammalian counterparts. Among these, the cytokines are essential effector molecules of innate and adaptive immunity against pathogenic microorganisms. Current dogma holds that cytokines are classified by the Thl-Th2 paradigm according to their role in the immune response (Mosmann & Coffman, 1989 & Degen *et al.*, 2005).

As in mammals, host inflammation and innate immunity in chickens are mediated by Th1 or Th1-related cytokines, including interferon (IFN)-α, -β and $-\gamma$, IL-1β, IL-2, IL-6, IL-10, IL-12, IL-15, IL-16, IL-17 and IL-18. In addition, other molecules such as myeloid differentiation factor 88 (MyD88), TNF receptor associated factor-5 (TRAF-5), and inducible nitric oxide synthase (iNOS) are involved in the Th1 inflammatory response to avian pathogens (Lin *et al.*, 1996 & Caldwell *et a1.*, 2005). The Th2 or Th2-related molecules, classically defined as driving humoral immunity, produce a distinct panel of cytokines, in particular IL-3, IL-4, IL-5, IL-13, granulocyte macrophage-colony stimulating factor (GM-CSF), and transforming growth factor (TGF)-β4 (Jakowlew *et al.*, 1988 & Avery *et al.*, 2004).

Table 7.1 : Classification of cytokines based on function

Classification	Examples
Proinflammatory	IL-1β, IL-6, IL-8
TH1	IFN-γ, IL-2, IL-18
Th2	-
Th3/Tr1	TGF-β
Others	IFN-α, IFN-β, IL-15, IL-16

Interferon-gamma (IFN-γ)

The interferon is protein, released by lymphocytes in response to the presence of the pathogens such as virus, bacteria, parasite or tumor cell. These proteins allow communication between cells to trigger the immune system's protective defenses that eliminate the pathogens. Depending upon the type of receptors, through which interferon proteins signal, these may be Interferon type I (binds to IFN-α receptor, e.g. IFN-β and IFN-ω; Interferon type II (binds to IFNGR, e.g. IFN-g; and Interferon type III (binds to a receptor complex consisting of IL10R2 and IFNLR1. The IFN-γ is also known as Immune interferon or macrophage activation factor.

IFN-γ gene

Interferon-γ gene sequences have been studied in 20 mammalian and five avian species. Comparison of the sequences among these different species reveals a highly conserved overall structure (Mehra, 2010a). The size of *IFN-γ* gene is 3.9kb in human and 2.9kb in chicken. The exon-intron structure shows considerable similarity in size and organization in mammals and avian (Kaiser *et al.*, 1998a). In all the species so far studied, it seems that IFN-γ is coded by a single copy gene. It has been mapped to chromosome chromosome 1 p24-p23 in chicken (Habermann *et al.*, 2001). Interferon-γ gene in mammals and birds has four exons. The third intron is the longest in mammals, whereas the second one is longest in chicken. IFN-γ gene sequence analysis has been done in different members of galliformis. The highly conserved structure of the gene and high degree of overall identity at the predicted primary amino acid sequence level of protein (including IFN-γ receptor binding motifs) suggest that IFN-γ may be cross reactive among these species (Kaiser *et al.*, 1998b).

The gene comprises four exons in chicken (Kaiser et al., 1998b). The first exon contains 5′ UTR and 123 nucleotides which codes for the signal sequence of 19 amino acid and the first 22 amino acid of the mature protein. Exons 2 and 3 comprised of 69 and 180 nucleotides, coding for 23 and 60 aa, respectively. Exon 4 comprised of 120 nucleotides coding for 40 aa, 3 nucleotides of stop codon and the 3′ UTR (>1278 bp).

In Indian RJF, size of the complete IFN-γ CDS was a 495 bp and no size variation was observed in nucleotide sequence (495 aa) as well as amino acid sequence (165 aa) between RJF and other poultry species including chicken.

Between RJF and other chicken breeds except very low polymorphism in nucleotide as well as amino acid sequence and most of this polymorphism was limited to Chinese Hui Yang breed. Between RJF and other poultry species, the polymorphism in nucleotide sequence ranged from 3.43 % between RJF and turkey to 19.39 between RJF & duck. In amino acid sequence, this range was from 3.03 between RJF and turkey to 32.73 between RJF & duck.

Structure of RJF IFN-γ gene: The genomic structure of the gene encoding the chicken homologue of IFN-γ was determined by Kaiser et al. (1998b). The gene comprises four exons. The first exon contains 5′ UTR and 123 nucleotides which codes for the signal sequence of 19 amino acid and the first 22 amino acid of the mature protein. Exons 2 and 3 comprised of 69 and 180 nucleotides, coding for 23 and 60 aa, respectively. Exon 4 comprised of 120 nucleotides coding for 40 aa, 3 nucleotides of stop codon and the 3′ UTR (>1278 bp).

The ORF of RJF IFN-γ encodes a polypeptide of 164 amino acids, of these, 41, 23, 60 and 40 amino acids are encode by exon 1, 2, 3 and 4 respectively (Mehra, 2010a). The deduced amino acid sequence of RJF IFN-γ was compared with those of other avian and mammalian species. The alignment analysis showed that Rjf IFN-γ shared 99.4 % homology with ChIFN-g, 97.0% identity with TuIFN-γ and 67% to 94% with other avian species whereas 20% to 30% identity with mammalian species. The highly conserved structure of the gene and high degree of overall identity at the predicted primary amino acid sequence level of protein has been reported within the species like Chicken (Anonymous, 2004) and duck (Huang et al., 2001).

Like HuIFN-γ protein, the Rjf IFN-γ mature protein exist as dimer of two identical subunits and each subunit consists of six helixes (Figure 7.1) Analysis of the signal peptide revealed that there was a potential cleavage site between amino acid residue 19 and 20. The mature RJF IFN-g appeared to consist of 145 amino acids and contained two cysteines located at amino acid residue143 and 145. Furthermore , two potential N-glycosylation sites were located in the protein similar to the chicken IFN-γ protein where as the duIFN-γ and the goIFN-γ protein has three sites, analysied with the NetNGlyc 1.0 server [http://www.cbs.dtu.dk/services/], suggesting that the Rjf IFN-γ, like other avian and mammalian type II IFNs, is a glycoprotein.

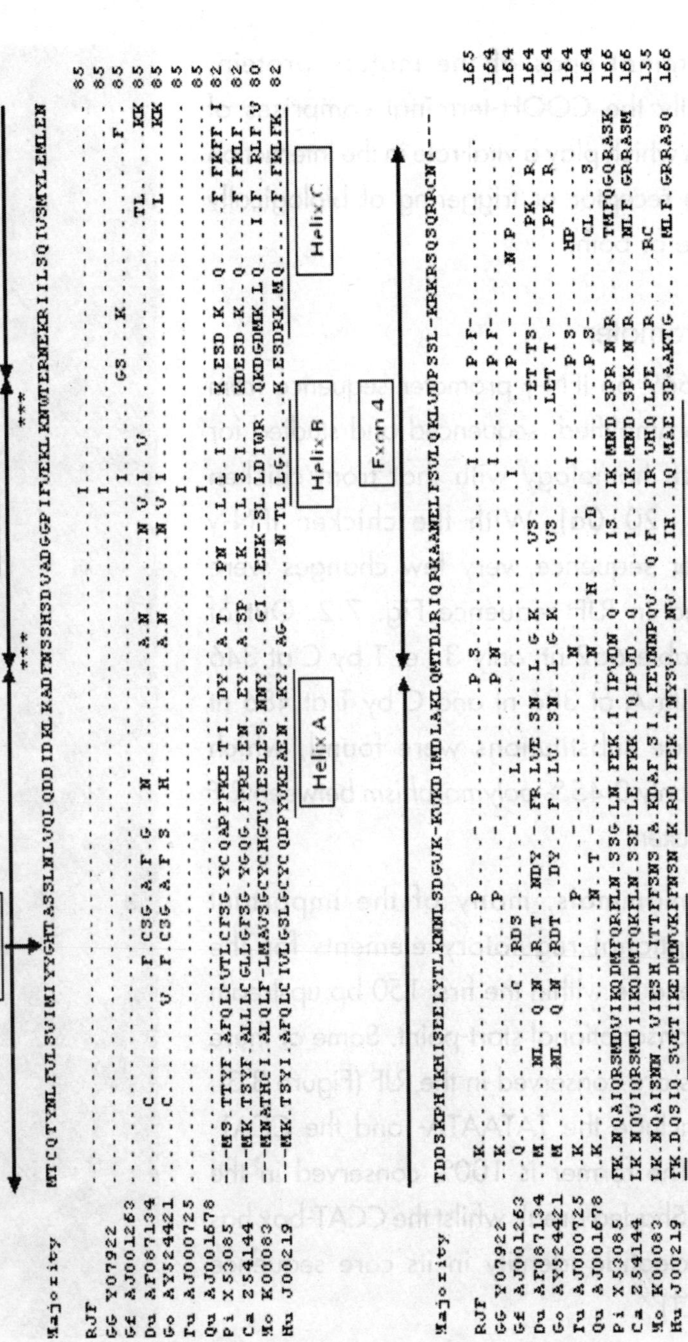

Fig. 7.1 : Structural and functional homology between IFN-γ CDS in RJF and other related species.

The terminal ends of the mature protein, especially the COOH-terminal comprises of residues which play a vital role in the interaction with the receptor or triggering of biologically response or both.

IFN- promoter

A 669 bp IFN-γ promoter sequence from RJF was amplified, sequenced and studied for sequence homology with that from chicken (Mehra, 2010a). With the chicken IFN-γ promoter sequence, very few changes were observed in RJF sequence Fig. 7.2. Out of comparable 662 nt, only 3 i.e. T by C at 346 nt, G with A at 386 nt and C by T at 486 nt nucleotide substitutions were found, which yielded only 0.45 % *polymorphism between RJF and chicken.*

In mammals, many of the important transcriptional regulatory elements for the IFN-γ gene lie within the first 150 bp upstream of the transcriptional start-point. Some of these elements are conserved in the RJF (Figure 8.3). These include the TATAATA- and the CCAT-boxes. The former is 100% conserved in the RJFken (Shaded area), whilst the CCAT-box has 3/6 nucleotide identity in its core sequence (CCATCT).

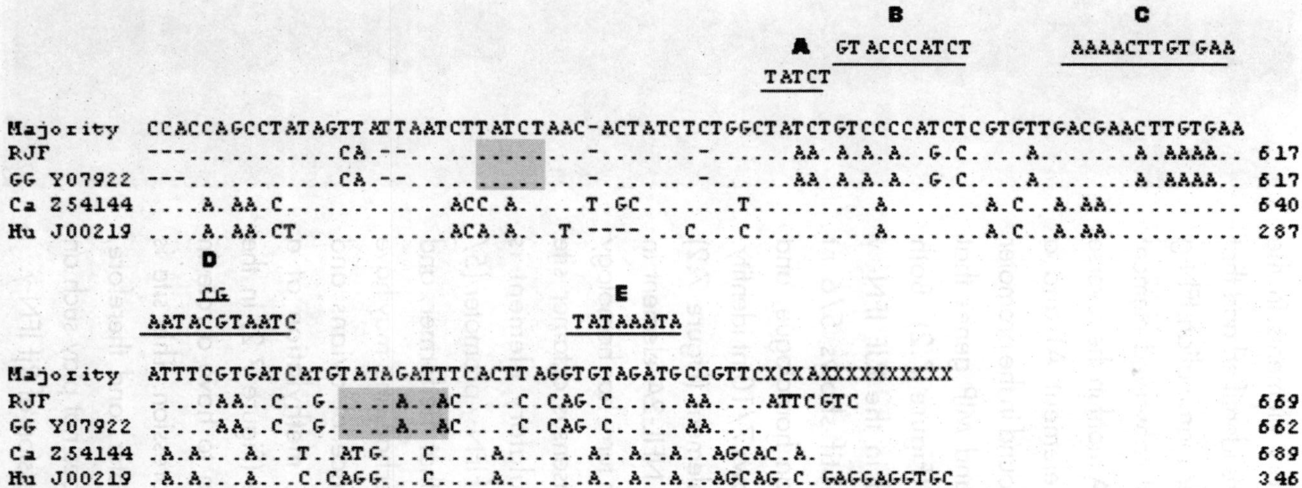

Fig. 7.2 : Structural and functional homology between IFN-γ promoter region in RJF and other related species. The putative transcriptional elements in the promoter, initially identified in other mammalian species by their homology with human and murine IFN-γ gene elements, are underlined.

Two essential regulatory elements in the human IFN-g promoter were identified and that are also conserved in other mammalian IFN-g gene promoters. The distal conserved element contains a consensus GATA motif in the reverse orientation (Fig. 2.20, element A) and a potential regulatory motif, found in the promoter regions of the GM-CSF and MIP genes that includes the CCAT-box (Figure 7.2). Both sequences are conserved in the RJF IFN- γ promoter. The GATA motif shows 5/6 nt identity with its mammalian homologue, and the GM-CSF/MIP motif shows 7/10 nt identity. The proximal conserved element (Figure 7.2) shares homology with the NFIL-2A element in the IL-2 promoter, which, in turn, has homology at its 3′ end with the consensus octamer site (ATGCAAAT). This regulatory element is apparently absent in the Rjf IFN-γ promoter (5/24 nt identity),suggesting that the former, and its associated regulatory mechanisms, may have arisen after the divergence of avians and mammals. In mammals, methylation at a conserved CpG target site (Figure 7.2) in the promoter has been shown to have a role in regulating IFN-γ gene expression. This site is absent in the IFN-γ promoter, and therefore, methylation presumably does not play such an important role in the expression of Rjf IFN-γ.

IFN- Receptor 2

A 674 bp of the Rjf IFN-γ receptor 2 gene was amplified, sequenced and studied for sequence homology with that from other related species (Mehra, 2010a). With the chicken IFN-γ R2 sequence, very few changes were observed in RJF sequence. Out of comparable 674 nt between RJF and chicken sequence, only 1 substitution i.e. A by G at 219 nt position was found and this substitution was transition. The 224 aa IFN-γ R2 sequence from RJF was compared with that from chicken. With the chicken IFN-γ R2 sequence, very few changes were observed in RJF sequence. Out of comparable 224 aa between RJF and chicken sequence, only 1 substitution i.e. N by D at 73 aa position was found.

In chicken the complete CDS of the IFN-γ R2 was 1005 bp which code for 335 amino acids. The IFN-γ R2 sequence in RJF was the partial and lacks 10 nt at 5′ end and 321 nt at 3′ end. Complete structural and functional homology was observed between comparable regions of IFN-γ R2 gene.

Interlukin-2 (IL-2)

Interleukin-2 or T-cell growth factor is one of the first cytokines to be characterized at molecular level. It is now considered as a central molecule of immune response. IL-2 is essential for maturation and growth of antigen specific B-and T-lymphocytes and for induction of other important cytokines from lymphocytes and macrophages.

IL2 gene

IL-2 gene is a single copy gene located on chromosome 4 in chicken. The size of IL-2 gene is approximately 4.4 kb in human, 4.166 kb in mice and 2.39 kb in chicken. IL-2 gene has four exons in human (Degrave *et al.*, 1983; Fujita *et al.*, 1983), in mice (Fuse *et al.*, 1984) and in chicken (Kaiser & Mariani, 1999). The major upstream regulatory elements are present in the region of –1 to –350. They are sites for binding of various transcription factors such as AP-1, NFkB and NF-AT. IL-2 promoters contain two NF-AT binding sites and one NFkB binding site (Garrity *et al.*, 1994). The NF-AT and AP-1 binding sites are highly conserved in mammalian and chicken IL-2 whereas, NFkB binding site is less conserved. The 3′ UTR of IL-2 contains 'ATTTA' instability motif, which mediate rapid mRNA degradation (Shaw & Kamen, 1986). Mammalian IL-2 and IL-2 from chicken and turkey have five such regions in their 3′UTR. Another functionally important sequence in the 3′UTR of IL-2 gene is the polyadenylation signal "AATAAA".

The IL-2 gene is composed of four exons and 3 introns in chicken (Kaiser and Mariani, 1999). A 432 bp fragment was amplified by using cDNA as template in Indian RJF and sequenced (Mehra, 2010a). This 432 bp sequence represented the complete CDS and codes for 141 amino acids sequence. For amino acid sequences, while no size variation was observed between RJF and chicken lines/ breeds (except AY766163 in which the aa sequence was 142 aa in size), the complete CDs was 142, 144, 140, 140 and 141 while in quail, turkey, duck, muscovy duck and goose, the sizes were, respectively. While between RJF and chicken very low polymorphism (2.08 %) was observed, much higher polymorphism (29.86 % to 38.57 %) was observed between RJF and other poultry species.

Structure of IL2 CDS: The 432 base pair fragments represent the complete coding region, comprising of Exon 1 to Exon 4 and comparison with chicken IL-2 sequence revealed that in RJF IL-2, Exon 1 is comprised of 22 aa of signal peptides and first 26 aa of mature peptide whereas exon 2, 3 and 4 encode 13, 46 and

36 aa respectively. These results suggest that rjflL-2 is exactly similar to chicken IL-2 (Kaiser and Muriani, 1999) in size and exonic structure. However, in other poultry species, the while Turkey IL-2 had the coding region of 143 aa, in duck and quail it was 140 aa and 142 aa, respectively (Shreekumar et al., 2005), whereas in goose, it was 141 aa (Zhou et al., 2003).

The amino acid sequence of Rjf IL-2 was aligned with IL-2 sequences from different poultry species as well as mammalian species (Figure 7.3). RJF showed a very high percentage amino acid identity with chicken (97.2%) indicating a high functional and structural similarity, while in other poultry species the percentage amino acid variability range from 60.3% (duck) to 72.9% (turkey). From there mammalian counterparts, amino acid variability ranges from 9.0% (sheep) to 15.3% (human). Earlier reports also revealed very low similarity between chicken and human IL2 (Kaiser and Muriani, 1999, Shreekumar et al., 2003) and goose IL2 and human (Jhou et al., 2003)

The deletions of 2 aa, 9 aa, and 1 aa between Thr^{19}- Ala^{20}, Lys^{49}- Ile^{50}, and Lys^{126}-Phe^{127}, respectively were found in RJF IL-2 in comparison to the mammalian IL2-CDS and these deletions were well conserved in all poultry species.

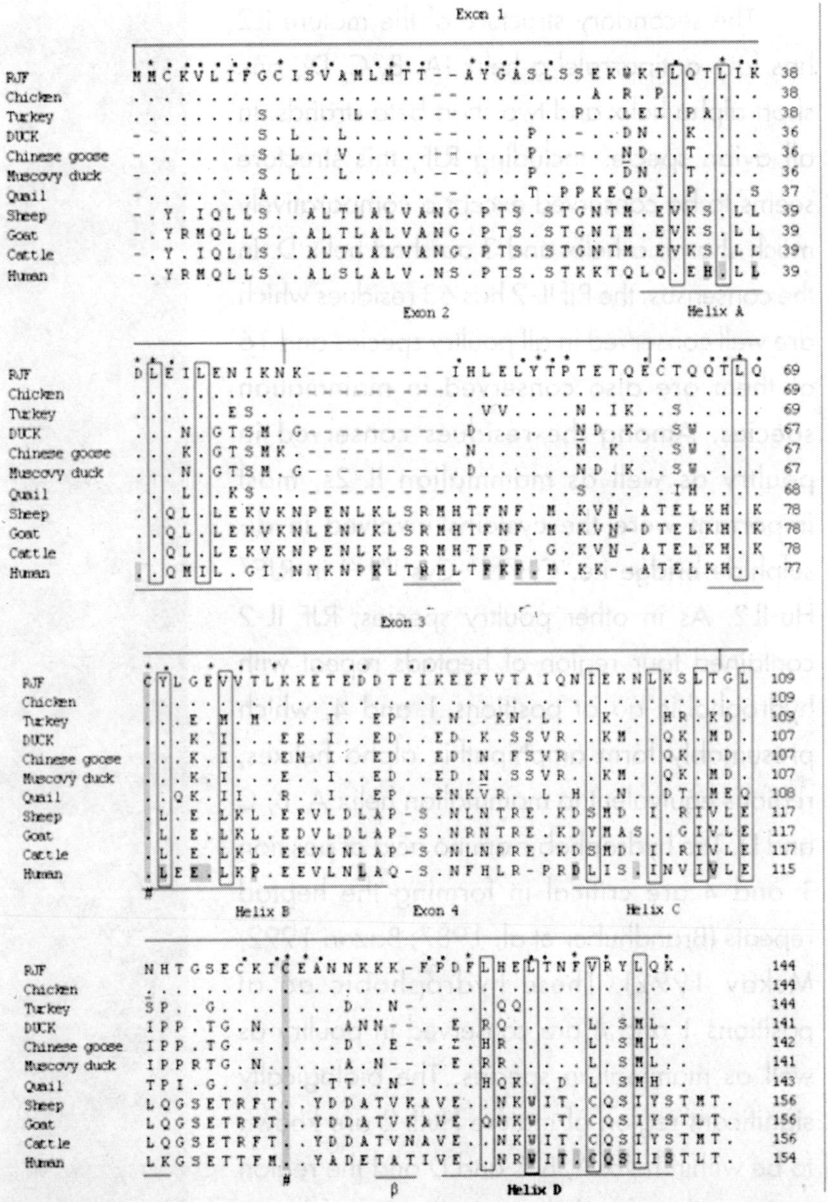

Fig. 7.3 : Structural and functional homology between IL2 CDS of RJF and other related species.

The secondary structure of the mature IL2 has four antiparralel a helix (A, B, C, D), one short alpha helix and two short beta strands. In all avian species including RJF, this structure seems to be conserved except a comparatively much shorter a helix and 3 aa short helix D. In the consensus, the Rjf IL-2 has 63 residues which are well conserved in all poultry species and 16 of them are also conserved in mammalian species. Among the residues conserved in poultry as well as mammalian IL-2s, most important were the cysteins involved in disulphide bridge i.e. $Cys^{70(78)}$-$Cys^{119(125)}$ in RJF/Hu-IL2. As in other poultry species, RJF IL-2 contained four region of heptads repeat with hydrophobic aa at positions 1 and 4, which presumably form amphipathic alpha helixes, regions equivalent to mammalian helix A, B, C and D. The hydrophobic amino acid at position 1 and 4 are critical in forming the heptad repeats (Brandhuber et al, 1987; Bazan 1992; Mckay 1992). These hydrophobic aa at positions 1 and 4 are conserved in poultry as well as mammalian species. The biologically significant region of mature HuIL-2 are known to be within helix A, B C and D and the region spanning between helix A and B. Out of the 25 residues involved in binding of IL2 receptors,

20 residues (80 %) were conserved between HuIL2 and IL2 from lives stock species, while only 6 i.e. Leu^{37},Asp^{40}, Tyr^{65}, Glu^{82}, Asn^{108}, Phe^{144} were conserved between HuIL2 and IL2 from poultry species including RJF and these residues were also conserved in live stock species.

IL-2 promoter gene

The 658 bp sequence amplified in RJF was comprised of initial 71 nt of exons and 587 nucleotides upstream the start code of signal peptide (Mehra, 2010a). Similarly in chicken, the IL2 promoter region sequence was of 650 bp upstream the start codon of signal peptide. The Rjf IL-2 promoter sequence showed very high sequence homology with that from chicken as among the comparable 587 nucleotides, only two nucleotide substitutions (0.30%) were observed, while comparatively higher polymorphism was observed between the comparable nucleotides, ranging from 2.97% between RJF and turkey to 10.05 between RJF and duck.

Structure of IL – 2 promoter gene: A 658 bp fragments of Rjf IL-2 promoter sequence was amplified from genomic DNA. This amplified region has the initial 71 nt of exon 1 which includes 66 nt of signal peptide and 5 nt of mature peptide which established the continuities of amplified region with the IL-2 cDNA. The 5′ UTR of RJF is small (63 nt) as also in other poultry species including chicken and human. In RJF IL-2 promoter sequence the putative transcription factors binding elements were identified by comparing it with chicken and human IL-2 prometer sequences. All the essential transcription factors binding sites identified in chicken (such as CD28 RE, NF KB, NF-AT and AP-1) were conserved in RJF IL-2 promoter also (Figure 7.4).

The potential proximal NF-AT, CD28 RE, TATA Box and distal AP-1 sites shows 100 % identity with chicken and human homologus. While proximal AP-1 shows 6/6 nt, 5/6 nt identity, NF-KB shows 11/11 nt, 4/11nt identity and distal NF-AT shows 10/10 nt, 9/10 nt identity with chicken and human IL-2 promoter sequences respectively. Like in chicken IL-2 promoter sequence (Kaiser and Mariani, 1999), two octomer binding site are almost absent in Rjf IL-2 promoter sequence. A high degree of identity was observed between RJF, poultry species and humans in the transcriptional initiation region.

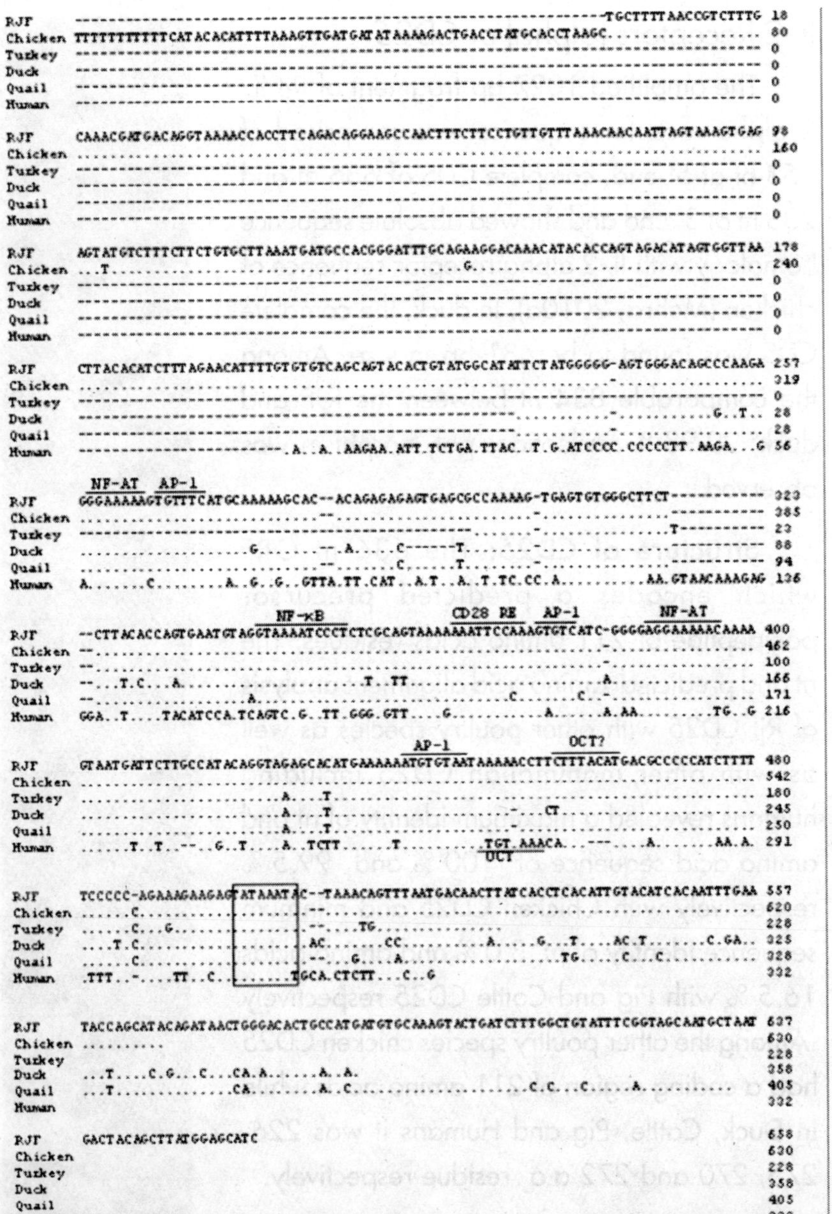

Fig. 7.4 : Structural and functional homology between IL2 promoter region in RJF and other related species

IL-2 Receptors (alpha) or CD25

The amplified 1027 bp fragment of Rjf IL-2 alpha receptor sequence was comprised of 153 nt at 5′ end, complete CDS of 636 nt and 238 nt at 3′ end and showed absolute sequence homology with IL-2 alpha receptor sequence of chicken (Mehra, 2010a). In duck, the complete CDS was found to be 681 bp in size. Among the comparable 834 nt between the RJF and duck, 20.98 % nucleotides polymorphism was observed.

Structure of CD25: The 636 nt ORF which encodes a predicted precursor polypeptide of 211 amino acids residues. The nt and predicted amino acid alignment analysis of Rjf CD25 with other poultry species as well as with other mammalian CD25 including humans revealed a maximum identity of nt and amino acid sequence of 100 % and 99.5 % respectively with Chicken CD25 and minmum sequence identity of nt 3.0 % and amino acids 16.5 % with Pig and Cattle CD25 respectively .Among the other poultry species chicken CD25 had a coding region of 211 amino acids while in Duck, Cattle, Pig and Humans it was 226, 275, 270 and 272 a.a residue respectively.

Signal peptide analysis revealed that the Rjf CD25 precursor polypeptide comprised of a signal peptide with 20 amino acids residue at the N- terminus. Further bioinformatics analysis showed that the predicted mature Rjf CD25 protein was composed of an extracellular domain (172 amino acid) a membrane spanning region (15 amino acid) and a cytoplasmic domain (4 amino acids). The Rjf CD25 contains 6 potential N-Gycolation sites (Figure 7.5) among the compared species. In the consensus, the Rjf CD 25 has 130 amino acids well conserved in all poultry species of which 35 amino acid are well conserved in all consensus species.

Especially the HuCD25 (Ref ASS.No. NP_000408) contains 5 di-sulphide bonds. Cys^{24}-Cys^{67}, Cys^{49}-Cys^{80}, Cys^{51}-Cys^{82}, Cys^{125}-Cys^{168} and Cys^{152}-Cys^{184}. Out of these 10 Cys residue 8 (at position Cys 23, 49, 65, 81, 121, 148, 164 & 180) are well conserved in RJF CD25 as well as in other compared poultry species, presumably allowing the formation of four di-sulphide bond in Rjf CD25. The amino acid residue Leu^{23}, Met^{46}, Leu^{63}, Tyr^{64}, Lys^{59}, Arg^{57}, Glu^{22}, Asp^{27} & Glu^{50} in HuCD25 are been implicated in IL-2 gene binding for the formation of IL-2/CD25 complex. Among these biologically significant amino acid residue Leu^{23}, Met^{46}, Tyr^{64}, Lys^{59}, and Glu^{20} have been

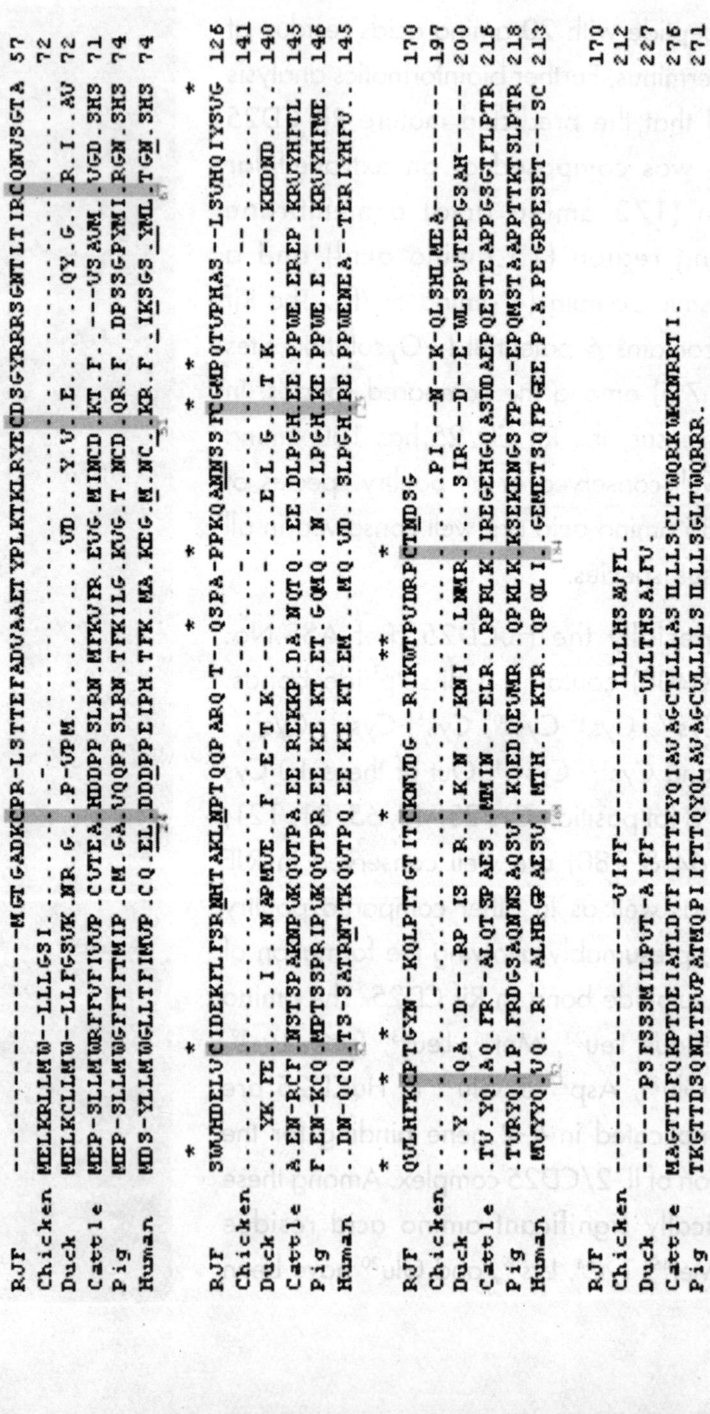

Fig. 7.5 : Structural and functional homology between CD25 region in RJF and other related species

substituted by Lys^{22}, Lys^{44}, Thr^{62}, Ser^{57} and Asp^{21} respectively in Rjf CD25 where as Lec^{63}, Arg^{57} and Glu^{50} residues are conserved while Asp^{27} has been deleted in Rjf CD25. However these changes did not affect the predicted conformation.

Interleukin 1-β (IL1-β)

Interleukin-1 (IL-1) is an important pro-inflammatory cytokine that exhibits pleiotropic activities on a wide range of target cells (Dinarello,1994). It is secreted by many different cell types, with stimulated macrophages being the main producers of IL-1.

RjfIL1- β

A 826 bp of IL1-β gene was amplified, sequenced in Indian RJF and studied for sequence homology comparison with that from related poultry species (Mehra, 2010b). Comparison of the rjf- IL1-β CDS with known chicken IL1-β showed that the 826 rjf- IL1-β is comprised 9 bp of 5′ UTR, complete exon 1 (41 nt), exon 2 (49 nt), exon 3 (184 nt), exon 4 (171 nt), exon 5 (146 nt), exon 6 (213 nt) and 13 nt of 3′ UTR. Therefore, the 826 bp includes complete CDS of 804 bp. A protein sequence of 267 amino acid, which includes a mature peptide of 162 amino acids, was predicted from this 804 nt complete CDS sequence.

Amino acid sequence variation: The amino acid sequence of IL-1β in red jungle fowl was 267 aa in size and it represented complete propeptide, Size of IL-1β propetide in chicken as well as other poultry species, was also 267 aa. Between the red jungle fowl and poultry species, percent sequence variability ranged from 0.75 % to 5.99 %. While red jungle fowl, it showed least sequence variability (0.75 %) with chicken as well as duck, much higher variability was observed with turkey (5.99 %). Size of Bovine and human IL-1β propetides were 266 aa and 269 aa, respectively and the percent sequence variability ranged from 67.47 to 68.16 between the red jungle fowl and mammals.

Structure of RjfIL-1β

The exonic structure of the IL-1â in mammals including livestock species (such as cattle, pig) and chicken is well defined (Bensi et al. 1987, Kaiser et al. 2004). In chicken, the size of IL-1β gene was found to be 1650 bp against the 7451 in human and 7069 in pig, however similar to its mammalian counterpart, it has six exons. Further perusal revealed that the much lower size of IL-1β gene in chicken is due to very small introns in comparison to their mammalian counterpart (Figure 7.6).

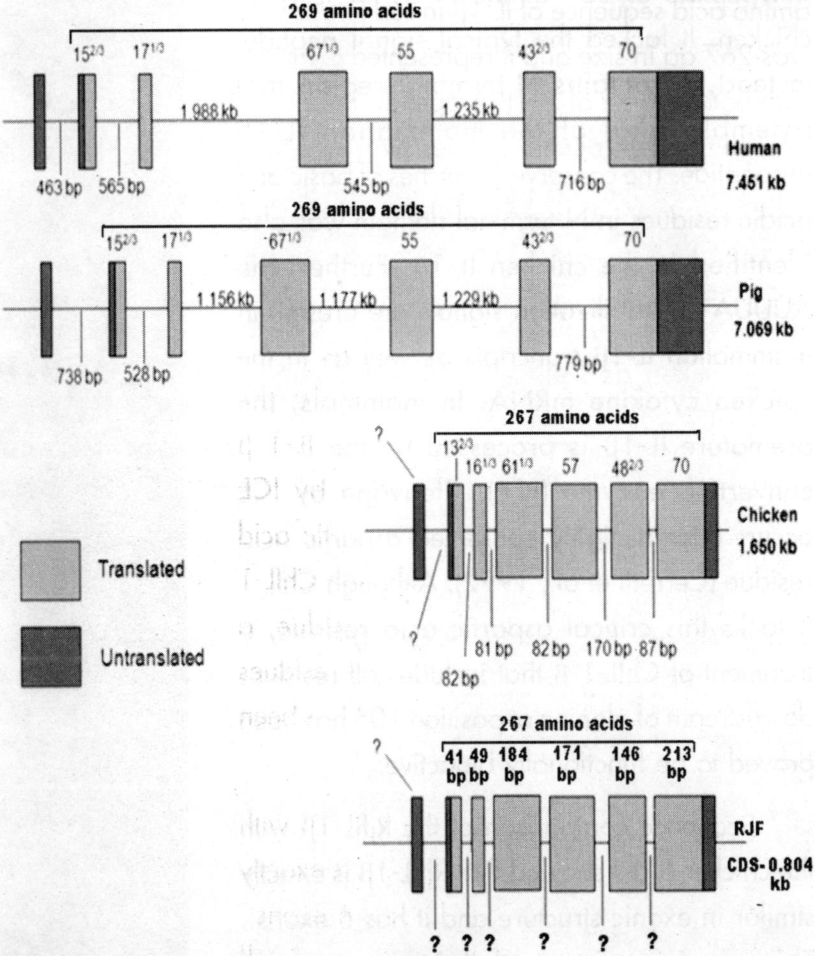

Fig. 7.6 : Comparison of IL1-β structure in RJF and chicken and the mammalian counterparts.

The size of IL-1β CDS was estimated to be 804 bp in chicken (Weining et al., 1998, Kaiser et al., 2004). Weining et al. (1998) characterized IL-1β in chicken. They reported a long open reading frame that codes for a polypeptide of 267 amino acids for IL-1β in chicken. It lacked the typical signal peptide. Instead, it contains N-terminal region that resembles that of the mammalian IL-1β propeptide. The conserved stretches of basic and acidic residues in N-terminal domain was also identified in the chicken IL-1β. Further, the AUUUA de-stabilization signals are present in mammalian IL-1β trancripts as well as in the chicken cytokine mRNA. In mammals, the premature IL-1β is processed by the IL-1 β converting enzyme (ICE). Cleavage by ICE occurs after a highly conserved aspartic acid residue (Cerretti et al., 1992). Although ChIL-1 β lacks this critical aspartic acid residue, a fragment of ChIL-1 β that includes all residues downstream of alanine at position 106 has been proved to be functionally bioactive.

Sequence comparison of the RjfIL-1β with the chicken IL-1β showed that RjfIL-1β is exactly similar in exonic structure and it has 6 exons.. This exonic structure of IL-1β is very well conserved in avian species. Sequence alignment of IL-1β among avian species revealed no size difference in CDS region among different poultry species .The proteolytic cleavage site for propeptide of mammalian IL-1β after a highly conserved aspartic acid residue, which was absent in chicken, was also lacked in rjf-IL1β (Figure 7.7). This feature was very well conserved across all the poultry species. The absence of this cleavage site was also observed in IL-1β of other non-mammalian species like catshark, crab, trout etc (Bird et al., 2002).

```
                      111111111122222222223333333333444444444455555555556
             -1234567890123456789012345678901234567890123456789012345678901234567890
                      β1            β2        β3                  β4
                   =========    ======    =======          ========
mat-pep-rjf  -APAFRYTRSQSFDIFDINQKCFVLESPTQLVALHLQGPSSSQKVRLNIALYRPRGPRGSA
mat-pep-chk  -............................................................
Bovine       D----APVQ.IKCKLQ.RE..SL..A..CV.K....LSQEMNRQ.VFCMSFVQ-----.EE
Human        D----APV..LNCTLR.SQ..SL.MSG.YE.K.....QDME.Q.VFSMSFVQ-----.EE
             Δ
                                                    11111111111111111111
             666666666677777777778888888888999999999900000000001111111112
             123456789012345678901234567890123456789012345678901234567890
                 B5            β6           β7                 β8
               ===========  =========   =========          ========
mat-pep-rjf  GTGQMP-VALGIKGYKLYMSCVMSGTEPTLQLEEADVMRDIDSVELTRFIFYRLDSPTEG
mat-pep-chk  .....-......................................................
Bovine       RDNKI.P......DKN..L...KK.DT.......V.PKVYPKRNMEK..V..KTEIKN--
Human        SNDKI.-....L.EKN..L...LKDDK......SV.PKNYPKKKMEK..V.NKIEINN--
             111111111111111111111111111111111111111111111
             222222222233333333334444444444555555555566666
             123456789012345678901234567890123456789012345
                B9          β10      β11           β12
             =======    ======   =======     ==========
mat-pep-rjf  TTRFESAAFPGWFICTSLQPRQPVGITNQPNQVNIATYKLS----
mat-pep-chk  ...............................D.........GR--
Bovine       .VE...VLY.N.Y.S..QIEER..FLGHFRAGQD.TDFRMETLSP
Human        KLE....Q..N.Y.S..QAENM..FLGGTKGGQD.TDFTMQFVSS
```

Fig. 7.7 : Alignment of the IL-1β amino acid sequence of RJF with chicken and mammalian species. "-" : gaps in the sequences; "." same amino acid as in RJF, = : beta strand; D: Highly conserved aspartate residue present in mammalian IL-1β, after which propeptides are cleaved.

From the 804 nucleotides of RjfIL-1 β, a pro-peptide of 267 amino acid was predicted which include mature peptide of 162 amino acids. Complete mature peptide was of 162 amino acids in chicken also. The mature IL-1β polypeptides from other poultry species were also have 162 amino acids, suggesting highly conserved size of mature IL-1B peptide. Wu et al. (2007) also reported that IL-1β encoding region of chicken, duck, goose and turkey was 804 bp, coding for IL-1β protein of 268 amino acids. The mature IL1β peptide amino acid sequences from RJF as well as from other poultry species including chicken (Figure 7.8) showed that the region that would be expected to represent the 12 β sheets is absolutely conserved in all the poultry species except turkey.

Interleukin-8 (IL-8)

IL-8 is a powerful chemotactic factor for neutrophils and was the first identified "chemokine". Macrophages and endothelial cells secrete IL-8 when stimulated by IL-1, TNF-α for bacterial products in order to attract neutrophils and allow them to adhere to vascular endothelial cells. This helps the neutrophils marginate on local blood vessels and enter the tissue where they are needed at sites of

```
                      111111111122222222223333333333444444444455555555556
             123456789012345678901234567890123456789012345678901234567890
             ♦                   •
                        β1         β2       β3            β4
                    =========   ======  ========      =========
HM179638-RJF APAFRYTRSQSFDIFDINQKCFVLESPTQLVALHLQGPSSQKVRLNIALYRPRGPRGSA
Y15006-CDS   ............................................................
AJ245728_Ck  ............................................................
DQ393268_Dk  ............................................................
DQ393269_Gs  ............................................................
DQ393271_Tuk ............................................................
                                                   1111111111111111111111
             666677777777778888888888999999999999999900000000001111111112
             123456789012345678901234567890123456789012345678901234567890
                                •
                    B5         β6         β7                    β8
               ==========  =========   =========            ========    =
HM179638-RJF GTGQMPVALGIKGYKLYMSCVMSGTEPTLQLEEADVMRDIDSVELTRFIFYRLDSPTEGT
Y15006-CDS   ............................................................
AJ245728_Ck  ............................................................
DQ393268_Dk  ............................................................
DQ393269_Gs  ..........................................................C.
DQ393271_Tuk .A..T................L..A...........T.....A.....V.......A...
             111111111111111111111111111111111111111111
             222222222333333333344444444445555555555666
             123456789012345678901234567890123456789012
                          •
               B9         β10      β11           β12
             ======   ======   ========     ===========
HM179638-RJF TRFESAAFPGWFICTSLQPRQPVGITNQPNQVNIATYKLS--
Y15006-CDS   ..............................D.........GR
AJ245728_Ck  ..............................D.........GR
DQ393268_Dk  ..............................D.........GR
DQ393269_Gs  ..............................D.........GR
DQ393271_Tuk ............................R.D.........GR
```

Fig. 7.8 : Alignment of the IL-1β amino acid sequence of RJF with five avian species. "-" : gaps in the sequences; "." Residues same as in RJF; = : residues involved in â strand formation; ¨ : Alanine confirmed as the start of the mature IL-1â and is conserved among all the species; • : Cysteine residues.

inflammation and infection. Interleukin-8 (IL-8) is a member of the chemokines which is structurally related to cytokines with chemotactic activity (Baggiolini *et al.*, 1997).

Most chemokines consist of four conserved cysteines which are important for their tertiary structures. Based on the spacing between the first two cysteines, chemokines can be subgrouped into CXC, CC, or CX3C subfamilies. In the chicken a number of CXC and CC chemokines have been identified (Kaiser *et al.*, 1999; Hughes and Bumstead, 2000, Hughes *et al.*, 2001). As in man, the CXC chemokine genes of the chicken are clustered on chromosome 4 (Kaiser *et al.*, 1999; Hughes and Bumstead, 2000). The chicken chemokine IL8/CAF appears to be the equivalent of mammalian IL-8. Originally termed 9E3/CEF4, this chemokine was the first non-mammalian cytokine cDNA to be cloned (Bedard *et al.*, 1987: Sugano *et al.*, 1987).

Kaiser *et al.* (1999) reported that the genomic structure of this gene is remarkably similar to one group of mammalian CXC cytokine genes; the gene comprises four exons and three introns. The first exon contains 5b UTR (un-translated region), a signal sequence of 15/16 aa, and the first few aa of the mature protein. Exons 2-4 determine the rest of the coding region, and exon 4 also encodes the stop codon and the 3′ UTR. Exons 2 and 3 of the 9E3/CEF4 gene, which encode the core of the protein, are identical in size to exons 2 and 3 of human IL8. Overall, of the mammalian CXC cytokine genes, this structure is most like human IL8. First and third introns are similar in size to most mammalian CXC cytokine genes, but the second intron is larger.

RjfIL-8 gene

A 642 bp of IL8 gene was amplified, sequenced in Indian RJF and studied for sequence homology comparison with that from related poultry species (Mehra, 2010b). Comparison of the rjf-IL8 CDS with known chicken IL8 showed that the 642 bp Rjf-IL8 is comprised 20 bp of 5′ UTR, complete exon 1 (61 nt), exon 2 (136 nt), exon 3 (84 nt), exon 4 (31 nt) and 310 nt of 3′ UTR. Therefore, the 642 bp sequence of IL-8 includes complete CDS of 312 bp. A protein sequence of 103 amino acid was predicted from this 312 nt complete CDS sequence.

Amino acid sequence variation: The amino acid sequence of IL8 in red jungle fowl was 103 aa in size and it represented complete peptide. Size of IL8 petide in chicken as well as other poultry species, was also 103 aa. Between Indian RJF and other jungle fowls, there was absolute sequence. Similarly, there was absolute sequence homology between Indian RJF and chicken. Between Indian RJF and duck, 10 amino acids (9.71 %) were polymorphic, while between RJF and goose, 8 amino acids were polymorphic (7.77 %). Between RJF and turkey, 1 amino acid (0.97 %) and between RJF and guinea fowl, 2 amino acids (1.94 %) were polymorphic.

Structure of RjfIL-8

The exonic structure of IL-8 in chicken was described by Kaiser et al., (1999). They reported that there are four exons in chicken IL-8 gene (Figure 7.9). The exon 1 includes 75 nucleotides of 5′UTR and 61 nucleotides of coding region, whereas as exon 2 and 3 are 136 and 84 nucleotides in size. Exon 4 is comprised of 31 nucleotides of coding region and 733 nucleotides long 3′ UTR. Thus, the complete coding region in chicken IL-8 is 312 nucleotides long. This exonic structure was very well conserved in RjfIL-8.

Comparisons of the RjfIL-8 with those from other jungle fowls as well as other poultry species (Figure 7.10) that all IL-8 sequences contains four cysteines and a typical chemokine CXC motif at positions 33–35 (CQC), which is a general feature for IL-8 protein. Amino acid residues ELR motif immediately preceding the first cysteine residue, which were shown to involve in receptor binding in human IL-8 (Hebert et al., 1991; Kaiser et al., 1999), were conserved in IL-8 all of these avian species. Wu et al. (2008b) also reported that these features are very well conserved in five avian species i.e. chicken, duck, goose, turkey and pigeon.

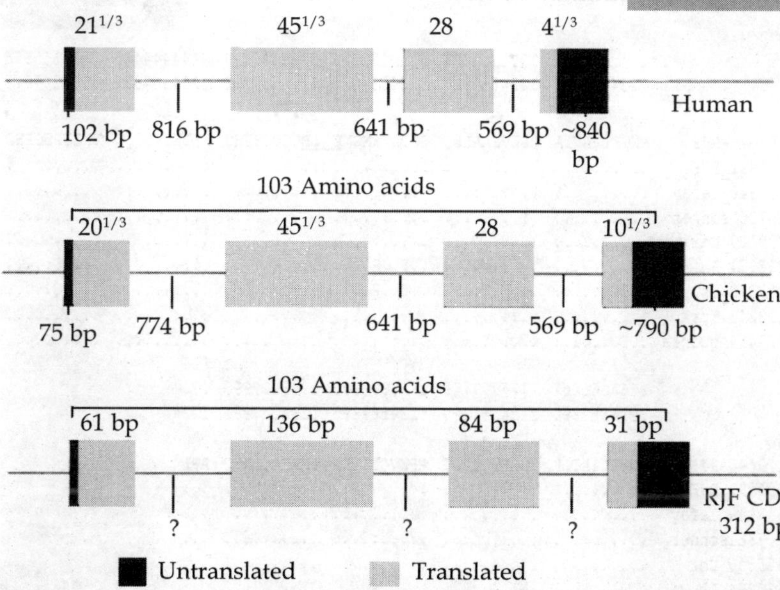

Fig. 7.9 : Comparison of IL-8 structure in RJF and chicken and the mammalian counterparts.

IL6 gene

Interleukin-6 (IL-6) is a multifunctional cytokine that plays a major role in regulating immune responses, acute phase reactions and haematopoiesis (Kishimoto *et al.*,1995). The IL-6 is the member of IL-6 family of cytokines which also includes IL-11, ciliary neurotrophic factor (CNTF), leukemia inhibitory factor (LIF), oncostatin M (OSM) and cardiotrophin-1 (Cr-1). These proteins share a common helical structure with four anti-parallel a helices, and act via a common signal transuding receptor chain (gp130) (Bazan 1990).

```
                         1 1111111112 2222222223 3333333334 4444444445 5555555556
                1234567890 1234567890 1234567890 1234567890 1234567890 1234567890
                                                   • •                          •
HM179640-RJF    MNGKLGAVLA LLLVSAALSQ GRTLVKMGNE LRCQCISTHS KFIHPKSIQD VKLTPSGPHC
NC006091_RJF    .......... .......... .......... .......... .......... ..........
FJ907840_lafay  .......... .......... .......... .......... .......... ..........
FJ907861sonner  .......... .......... .......... .......... .......... ..........
AJ009800_Chk    .......... .......... .......... .......... .......... ..........
AB236334_Dk     ......V... ...I.V.... ..S..R.... .......... .......... ....Q.....
AB213393_Gs     .......... ...I.V.... ..S..R.... .......... .......... ....Q.....
DQ393276_Turk   .......... .......... .......... .......... .......... ..........
GQ227414_guinea ..S...I... .......... .......... .......... .......... ..........
                                                          1 111
                6666666667 7777777778 8888888889 9999999990 000
                1234567890 1234567890 1234567890 1234567890 123
                                •
HM179640-RJF    KNVEIIATLK DGREVCLDPT APWVQLIVKA LMAKAQLNSD APL
NC006091_RJF    .......... .......... .......... .......... ...
FJ907840_lafay  .......... .......... .......... .......... ...
FJ907861sonner  .......... .......... .......... .......... ...
AJ009800_Chk    .......... .......... .......... .......... ...
AB236334_Dk     .......... .N........ .....R.... IL........ ...
AB213393_Gs     .......... .N........ .......... IL........ ...
DQ393276_Turk   .......... .S........ .......... .......... ...
GQ227414_guinea .......... .......... .......... .......... ...
```

Fig. 7.10 : Alignment of the IL-8 amino acid sequence of RJF with avian species. "-" : gaps in the sequences; "." Residues same as in RJF; • : Cysteine residues. Amino acid sequences CQC (residues 33–35) which are general features for CXC chemokines are overlined. IL-8 receptor-binding residues (ELR) immediately preceding first cysteine residue of the CXC motif are underlined.

Coding region of the chicken IL6 gene consists of four exons and three introns (Kasier et al., 2004). Exons 1 and 2 in mammalian IL6 genes seem to be a single exon in the chicken IL6 gene. This presumably reflects intron loss in the chicken or intron gain in mammals. Complete chicken IL-6 (ChIL-6) open reading frame coded for a polypeptide of 241 amino acid residues (Figure 7.11). Sequence comparison with various IL-6 sequences of mammals revealed the presence of an unusually long signal peptide of 47 amino acids at the N-terminus of ChIL-6. Mature ChIL-6 thus appears to consist of 194 amino acids. The 3′ untranslated region consists of 394 nucleotides excluding the poly(A) tail. It harbors eight ATTTA sequence elements, typically found in cytokine mRNAs, which mediate RNA instability (Schneider et al., 2001).

RjfIL-6

A 762 bp of IL6 gene was amplified, sequenced in Indian RJF and studied for sequence homology comparison with that from related poultry species (Mehra, 2010b). Comparison of the Rjf-IL6 CDS with known chicken IL6 showed that the 762 bp Rjf-IL6 is comprised 13 bp of 5′ UTR (partial), complete exon 1 (273 nt), exon 2 (114 nt), exon 3 (147 nt), exon 4 (192 nt) and 23 nt of 3′ UTR (partial). Therefore, the 762 bp sequence of IL-6 includes complete CDS of 726 bp. First 141 nt codes for 47 AA long signal peptide, while remaining 132 nt codes for 44 AA of matured peptide. The exon 2, exon 3 and exon 4 codes for 38, 49 and 64 AA of mature peptide, respectively. Hence, overall a protein sequence of 241 amino acid was predicted from the 762 nt complete CDS sequence, which includes 47 AA of peptide signal and 194 AA of mature peptide.

Amino acid sequence variation: The amino acid sequence of IL6 in red jungle fowl was 242 aa in size and it represented 47 AA long signal peptide and 194 AA long mature peptide. Size of IL6 signal as well as mature peptide in chicken was same i.e. 47 AA long signal peptide and 194 AA long mature peptide. Among other poultry species, only partial mature peptide (127 AA) sequence was available in duck only. Between Indian RJF and chicken, out of 47 AA of signal peptide and 194 AA of mature peptide, only 1 AA (0.41 %) in mature peptide was found to be polymorphic. However among the 127 comparable AA of mature peptide between Indian RJF and Chicken, 13 (10.24 %) were polymorphic.

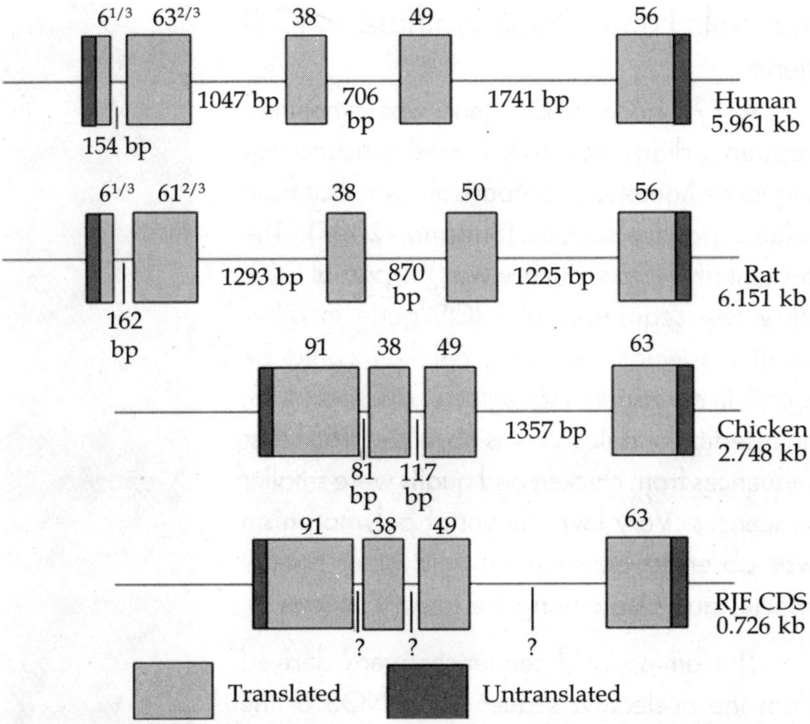

Fig. 7.11 : Comparison of IL16 structure in RJF and chicken and the mammalian counterparts.

Structure of RjfIL-6

Sequence homology comparison of RjfIL-6 with chicken IL-6 revealed very high degree of conservation in exonic structure between them. Hence, coding region of RjfIL-6 is 726 nucleotides in size, having four exons coding for 47 AA of signal peptide and 194 AA of mature peptide (Fig. 7.11). In other poultry species, only partial sequence of mature peptide is available, hence effective comparisons could not be made.

Inducible Nitric Oxide synthase (iNOS) gene

A 792 bp of iNOS gene was amplified, sequenced in Indian RJF and studied for sequence homology comparison with that from related poultry species (Sharma, 2007). The present rjf-iNOS sequence was the partial CDS. Very few sequences of iNOS gene in other poultry species including chicken could be found. In corresponding region of chicken iNOS, no insertion or deletion was observed. The other sequences from chicken and quails were smaller sequences. Very low amount of polymorphism was observed between RJF and other poultry species and also among the poultry species.

The amino acid sequences were derived from the nucleotide sequence of iNOS of the red jungle fowl as well as other poultry species and compared. The iNOS amino acid sequence comprised of 263 amino acid in RJF. The comparable sequence from chicken and guinea fowl also produced 263 aa, where as in quail, the available nucleotide sequence was partial and much smaller, hence produced only 123 amino acids. Out of 263 amino acids between red jungle fowl and chicken, only 1 site (0.4 %) was polymorphic, while number of polymorphic sites between RJF and guinea fowl as well as between guinea fowl and chicken were 6 (2.28 %) and 7 (2.66 %), respectively.

□□□

References

Ahmed, K.A., Saxena, V.K., Saxena, M., Ara, A., Pramod, A.B., Rajaram, M.L., Dorman, K.S., Majumdar, S. and Rasool, T.J. 2007. Molecular cloning and sequencing of MHC class II beta 1 domain of turkey reveals high sequence identity with chicken. International Journal of Immunogenetics 34, 97–105

Ahmed, S.U. 2009. Detection of single nucleotide polymorphism (SNP) in mitochondrial genome of Red Jungle Fowl (RJF) and its utilization in estimating of genetic diversity between RJF and domestic fowl Submitted to IVRI,Deemed University, Izatnagar

Anonymous 2004. Annual report 2003-2004, Central Avian Research Institute, Iztanagar, U.P., submitted to Central Library, Central Avian Research Institute, Iztanagar, U.P., India.

Avery, S., Rothwell, L., Degen, W.D., Schijns, V.E., Young, J., Kaufman, J. and Kaiser, P. 2004. Characterization of the first non-mammalian T2 cytokine gene cluster: the cluster contains functional single-copy genes for IL-3, IL-4, IL-13, and GM-CSF, a gene for IL-5 that appears to be a pseudogene and a gene encoding another cytokine like transcript, KK34. J. Interferon Cytokine Res. 24: 600-610.

Baggiolini, M., Dewald, B. and Moser, B., 1997. Human chemokines: an update. Annu. Rev. Immunol. 15, 675–705.

Baker, C.M.A., and C. Manwell, 1972. Molecular genetics of avian proteins. XI. Egg proteins of *Gallus gallus, G. sonnerati* and hybrids. Anim. Blood Grps. Biochem. Genet..3:101-107.

Baker, C.M.A., C. Manwell, N. Jayaprakash, and A.M. Francis, 1971. Molecular genetics of avian proteins - X. Egg white protein polymorphism of indigenous Indian chickens. Comp. Biochem. Physiol. 40B:147-153.

Bate, D.M.A., 1934. The domestic fowl in pre-Roman Britain. Ibis, series 13, 4:390-395.

Bazan, J. F. 1992. Unraveling the structure of IL-2. *Science* 257, 410-3.

Bazan, J.F. 1990. Structural design and molecular evolution of a cytokine receptor superfamily. Proc. Natl Acad. Sci. USA 87, 6934-6938.

Bedard, P.A., Alcorta, D., Simmons, D.L., Luk, K.C. and Erikson, R.L. 1987. Constitutive expression of a gene encoding a polypeptide homologous to biologically active human platelet protein in Rous sarcoma virus-transformed fibroblast. Proc. Natl. Acad. Sci. U.S.A. 84, 6715–6719.

Beebe, W., 1918-1922. A Monograph of Pheasants. Vols. I-IV. H.F. and G. Witherby, London.

Bensi, G., Raugei, G., Palla, E., Carinci, V., Tornese, B.D. and Melli, M. 1987. Human interleukin-1 beta gene. Gene 52 1, 95–101.

Bird, S., Wang, T., Zou, J., Cunningham, C. and Secombes, C.J. 2002. The First Cytokine Sequence Within Cartilaginous Fish: IL-1 {beta} in the Small Spotted Catshark Scyliorhinus canicula. J. Immunol. 168, 3329-3340.

Bokonyi, S., 1984. Animal Husbandry and Hunting in Tic-Gorsium. The Vertebrate Fauna of a Roman Town in Pannonia. Akademiai Kiado, Budapest.

Bourlet,Y., Behar,G., Guillemout,F., Frechin, N., Billault.A. and Chassee,A., 1988.Isolation of chicken major histocompatibility complex of class II B-L b chain sequences: comparison with mammalian beta chain and expression in lymphoid organs. EMBO Journal 7: 1031-1039

Brandhuber, B. J., Boone, T., Kenney, W. C. and McKay, D. B. 1987. Three-dimensional structure of interleukin-2. *Science* 238, 1707-1709.

Briles ,W., McGibbon, W. and Irwin, M. 1950. On multiple alleles affecting cellular antigens in the chicken. Genetics.35:633-640

Brown, E., 1906. Races of Domestic Poultry. Edward Arnold, London.

Brown, E., 1929. Poultry Breeding and Production. Vols. I & II. Ernest Benn Ltd., London.

Carter, G.F., 1971. Chapter 9 Pre-Columbian chickens in America. In: Riley, C.L., J.C. Kelley, C.W. Pennington, and R.L. Rands, editors. Man Across the Sea. Problems of Pre-Columbian Contacts. University of Texas Press, Austin.

Cerretti, D. P., Kozlosky, C. J., Mosley, B., Nelson, N., Van Ness, K., Greenstreet, T. A., March, C. J., Kronheim, S. R., Druck, T., Cannizzaro, L. A., Huebner, K. & Black, R. A. 1992. Molecular cloning of the interleukin-1beta converting enzyme. Science 256, 97-100.

Chow, B.S., 1984. Animal domestication in Neolithic China. In: Clutton-Brock, J., and C. Grigson, editors. Animals and Archaeology. Vol. 3: Early Herders and Their Flocks. British Archaeological Reports International Series 202.

Coltherd, J.B., 1966. The domestic fowl in ancient Egypt. Ibis 108:217-223.

Crawford, R.D., 1984. Chapter 42 Domestic fowl. Chapter 47 Turkey. Chapter 50 Goose. In: Mason, LL., editor. Evolution of Domesticated Animals. Longman Inc., New York.

Darwin CR (1868) The variation of animals and plants under domestication. London: John Murray.

Degen,W.G., Daal, N., Rothwell, L., Kaiser, P. and Schijns, V. E. 2005. Thl/Th2 polarization by viral and helminth infection in birds. Vet. Microbiol. 105: 163-167.

Degrave, W., Tavernier, J., Duerinck, F., Plaetinck, G., Devos, R. and Fiers, W. 1983. Cloning and structure of the human interleukin 2 chromosomal gene. Embo J 2, 2349-53.

Desjardins P and Morais R. 1991. Nucleotide sequence and Evolution of Coding and Noncoding Regions of a Quail Mitochondrial Genome. J Mol Evol 32 : 153-161.

Desjardins P. and Morais R. 1990. Sequence and gene organization of the chicken mitochondrial gene : a novel gene order in higher vertebrates. J Mol Biol 212 : 529-534.

Desjardins, P, Ramirez V and Morais, R. 1990. Gene organization of the Peking duck mitochondrial genome. Curr Genet 17 : 515-518.

Dinarello, C. A. 1994. Interleukin-1. In: *The Cytokine Handbook* Thompson, A., ed. p. 31, Academic Press, London.

Dodgson, J.B., Cheng, H.H. and Okimoto, R. (1997). DNA marker technology: A revolution in animal genetics. Poultry Science, 76: 1108-1114.

Douzery E and Randi E. 1997. The mitochondrial control region of Cervidae: evolutionary patterns and phylogenetic contents. Mol Biol Evol 14: 1154-1166.

Dufrense C, Mignotte F, Gueride M. 1996. The presence of tandem repeats and the initiation of replication in rabbit mitochondrial DNA. Eur J Biochem 235 : 593-600.

Eriksson J, Larson G, Gunnarsson U, Bed'hom B, Tixier-Boichard M, Stromstedt, L., Wright D, Jungerius A, Vereijken A, Randi E., Jensen P., Andersson, L. 2008. Identification of the yellow skin gene reveals a hybrid origin of the domestic chicken. PLoS Genet 4: e1000010. DOI: 10.1371/journal.pgen.1000010.

Ewald, S.J., Ye, X., Avendano, S., McLeod, S., Lamont, S.J. and Dekkers, J.C.M. 2007. Association of BF2 alleles with antibody titres and production traits in commercial pure line broiler population. Animal Genetics. 26 : 17326801.

Frisby, D.P., R.A. Weiss, M. Roussel, and D. Stehelin, 1979. The distribution of endogenous chicken retrovirus sequences in the DNA of galliform birds does not coincide with avian phylogenetic relationships. Cell 17:623-634.

Fu, Y., Niu, D., Luo, J., Ruan, H., He, G.Q. and Zhang, Y.P. (2001). Studies of the origin of Chinese domestic fowls. Yi Chuan Xue Bao. 28 (5) : 411-417.

Fujita, T., Takaoka, C., Matsui, H. and Taniguchi, T. 1983. Structure of the human interleukin 2 gene. Proc Natl Acad Sci U S A 80, 7437-41.

Fumihito, A., Miyake, T., Sumi, S., Takada, M., Ohno, S. and Kondo, N. 1994. One subspecies of the red junglefowl (Gallus gallus gallus) suffices as the matriarchic ancestor of all domestic breeds. Proc Natl Acad Sci U S A. 1994 Dec 20;91(26):12505-9.

Fumihito, A., Miyake, T., Takada, M., Shingu, R., Endo, T., Gojobori, T., Kondo, N. and Ohno, S. 1996. Monophyletic origin and unique dispersal patterns of domestic fowls. Proc Natl Acad Sci U S A. 1996 Jun 25;93(13):6792-5.

Fuse, A., Fujita, T., Yasumitsu, H., Kashima, N., Hasegawa, K. and Taniguchi, T. 1984. Organization and structure of the mouse interleukin-2 gene. *Nucleic Acids Res* 12, 9323-31.

Garrity, P. A., Chen, D., Rothenberg, E. V. and Wold, B. J. 1994. Interleukin-2 transcription is regulated in vivo at the level of coordinated binding of both constitutive and regulated factors. *Mol Cell Biol* 14, 2159-69.

Ghigi, A. 1916. Ricerche sull'incrociamento del Gallus sonnerati con polli domestici. Memorie della R. ccademia delle Scienze dell'Istituto diBologna, Classe di Scienze fisiche, 7th Ser., 3: 79–92.

Ghigi, A. 1922. L'hybridisme dans la génèse des races domestiques d'oiseaux. Genetica, 4: 364–374.

Goto, R., Miyada, C., Young, S., Wallace, R., Abplanalp, H., Bloom, S. and Brieles, W.E. 1988. Isolation of a cDNA clone from the B-G sub region of the chicken histocompatibility Bcomplex. Immunogenetics.102–109.

Guillemot, F., Billaut, A., Pourquie ,O., Behar ,A., Chasse ,A. and Zoorob, R. 1988.A molecular map of the chicken major histocompatibility complex; The class II b genes are closely linked to the class I genes and the nucleolar organizer.EMBO.J.7:2775-2785.

Habermann, F. A., Biet, C. and Fries, R. 2001. Chromosomal localization of the genes encoding SCNN1A, BTG1, IFNG and MAOA on chicken chromosome 1 by fluorescence in-situ hybridization. Chromosome Res 9, 515-8.

Hala, K., Palchy ,J. and Schulmannova ,J. 1981. Role of B- G antigen in the humoral immune response to the B- F antigen of chicken MHC. Immunogenetics, 14:393- 401.

Halushka, M.K., Fan, J.B., Bently, K., Hsie, L., Shen, N., Weder, A., Cooper,R., Lipshutz, R. and Chakravarti, A. 1999. Pattern of single nucleotide polymorphsms in candidate genes for blood-pressure homeostasis. Nat Genet., 22 : 239-247.

Harrison, C.J.O., 1978. A new jungle-fowl from the Pleistocene of Europe. J. Archaeol. Sci. 5:373-376. Hehn, V., 1885. The Wanderings of Plants and Animals from Their First Home. Swan Sonnenschein and Co., London.

Hertwig, P. 1936. Artbastarde bei Tieren.Handbuch der Vererbungswiss enschaft., 2 B (21).

Hillel, J., Groenen, M.A.M., Tixier Boichard, M., Korol, A.B., David, L., Kirzhner, V.M., Burke, T., Barre Dirie, A., Crooijmans, R.P.M.A., Elo, K., Feldman, M.W, Freidlin, P.J., Maki Tanila, A., Oortwijin, M., Thomson, P., Vignal, A., Wimmers, K., and Weigend, S. (2003). Biodiversity of 52 chicken populations assessed by microsatellite typing of DNA pools. Genetics, Selection, Evolution, 35(5): 553-557.

Ho, P.T., 1977. The indigenous origins of Chinese agriculture. In: Reed, C.A., editor. Origins of Agriculture. Mouton Publishers, The Hague.

Hosomichi,K., Shiina,T., Suzuki,S., Tanaka,M., Shimizu,S., Iwamoto,S., Hara,H., Yoshida,Y., Kulski,J.K., Inoko,H. and Hanzawa,K. 2006. The major histocompatibility complex Mhc class IIB region has greater genomic structural flexibility and diversity in the quail than the chicken. BMC Genomics 7:322.

Huang A., Scougall C.A., Lowenthal J.W., Jilbert A.R. and Kotlarski I. 2001. Structural and functional homology between duck and chicken interferon-gamma. Dev. Comp. Immunol. 25 1: 55-68.

Hughes S. and Bumstead, N. 2000. The gene encoding the chicken chemokine K60 maps to chromosome 4. Anim. Genet. 31, 418-419.

Hughes, S., Haynes, A., O'Regan, M. and Bumstead, N. 2001. Identification, mapping and phylogenetic analysis of three novel chicken CC chemokines. Immunogenetics. 58, 674-683.

Hunt, H.D. and Fulton, J.E. 1998. Analysis of polymorphism in the major expressed class I locus BFIV pf the chicken. Immunogenetics. 47 : 456-467.

Hyams, E., 1972. Animals in the Service of Man. 10,000 Years of Domestication. J.M. Dent & Sons Ltd., London.

Jakowlew, S.B., Dillard, P.J., Sporn M.B and Roberts, A.B. 1988. Complementary deoxyribonucleic acid cloning of a messenger ribonucleic acid encoding transforming growth factor beta 4 from chicken embryo chondrocytes. Mol. Endocrinol. 2: 1186-1195.

Jett, S.C., 1983. Chapter 12 Precolumbian transoceanic contacts. In: Jennings, J.D., editor. Ancient North Americans. W.H. Freeman and Company, San Francisco.

Kaiser, P. and Mariani, P. 1999. Promoter sequence, exon:intron structure, and synteny of genetic location show that a chicken cytokine with T-cell proliferative activity is IL2 and not IL15. Immunogenetics 49, 26-35.

Kaiser, P., Hughes, S. & Bumstead, N. 1999. The chicken 9E3/CEF4 CXC chemokine is the avian orthologue of IL8 and maps to chicken chromosome 4 syntenic with genes flanking the mammalian chemokine cluster. Immunogenetics 49., 673–84.

Kaiser, P., Rothwell, L., Goodchild, M. and Bumstead, N. 2004. The chicken proinflammatory cytokines interleukin-1b and interleukin-6: differences in gene structure and genetic location compared with their mammalian orthologues. Anim. Genet., 35, 169–175.

Kaiser, P., Sonnemans, D. and Smith, L. M. 1998a. Avian IFN-gamma genes: sequence analysis suggests probable cross-species reactivity among galliforms. J Interferon Cytokine Res 18, 711-9.

Kaiser, P., Wain, H. M. and Rothwell, L. 1998b. Structure of the chicken interferon-gamma gene, and comparison to mammalian homologues. Gene 207, 25-32.

Kanginakudru S, Metta M, Jakati RD and Nagaraju J. 2008. Genetic evidence from Indian red jungle fowl corroborates multiple domestication of modern day chicken. BMC Evolutionary Biology 8:174.

Kaufman, J., Milne ,S., Gobel ,T.W.F., Walker, R.A.1999 The chicken B locus is the minimal essential major histocompatibility complex. Nature 401:923-925.

Kim,H., Schmidt,C.J., Decker, K.S, Emara, M.G. 2002. Chicken SNP discovery by EST data mining, in : Plant, Animal & Microbe Genomes X, 12-16

January, San Diego, http:// www.intl-pag.org/ pag/10/ abstracts/ PAGX_p246.html.

Kishimoto, T., Akira, S., Narazaki, M. and Taga, T. 1995. Interleukin-6 family of cytokines and gp130. Blood 86, 1243-1254.

Komiyama, T., Ikeo, K., Tateno, Y., Gojobori, T., 2004. Japanese domesticated chickens have been derived from Shamo traditional Wghting cocks. Mol. Phylogenet. Evol. 33, 16–21.

Kumar Vinay (2010). Species specific DNA markers to monitor gene flow between Red Jungle Fowl (Gallus gallus) and domesticated chicken (Gallus gallus domesticus) Submitted to Bundelkhand University, Jhansi.

L'Abbe, L.D., Duhaime, J.F., Lang, B.F. Morais, R. (1991). The transcription of DNA in chicken mitochondria initiates from one major bidirectional promoter. J. Biol. Chem. 266(17): 10844-10850.

Laskowski, M., Kato, I., Ardelt, W., Cook, J., Denton, A., Empie, M. W., Khor, W. J., Park, S.J., Parks, K., Schatzely, B.L., Schoernberger, O.L., Tashiro, M., Vichot, G Whatley, H.E., Wieczcorek, A. & Wieczcorek, M.1987. Ovomucoid third domain form 100 avian species: Isolation, Sequencing and hypervariability of enzyme-inhibitor contact residues. Biochemistry, 26,202-21,

Lima-Rosa, C.A.V., Canal, C.W., Streck, A.F., Freitas, L.B., Delgado-Canedo, A., Bonatto, S.L. and Salzano et al. 2004. B-F DNA sequence variability in Brazilian blue egg Caipira chicken. Animal Genetics. 35 : 278-284.

Lind, L.R., translator, 1963. Aldrovandi on Chickens. The Ornithology of Ulisse Aldrovandi Volume II, Book XIV. University of Oklahoma Press, Norman.

Liu YP, Wu GS, Yao YG, Miao YW, Luikart G, Baig M., Beja-Pereira A., Ding, Z., Palanichamy M.G., Zhang, Y.P. 2006. Multiple maternal origins of chickens: out of the Asian jungles. Mol Phylogenet Evol 38: 12–19.

Lowe, P.R., 1934. A further note bearing on the date when the domestic fowl was first known ancient Egyptians. Ibis, series 13, 4:378-382.

Marshall HD and Baker AJ. 1997. Structural Conservation and Variation in the Mitochondrial Control Region of Fringilline Finches Fringilla spp. and the Greenfinch Carduelis chloris. Mol Biol Evol 14: 173-194.

McKay, D.B. 1992 Unraveling the structure of IL-2: response. Science, 257, 412.

Mehra, Somesh 2010. Comparative genomic studiesin Red Jungle Fowl (Gallus gallus gallus) and domesticated chicken. Submitted to Bundelkhand University, Jhansi.

Miller, M.M., Bacon, L.D., Hala, K., Hunt, H.D., Ewald, S.J., Kaufman, J., Zoorob, R., Briles, W.E.2004. Nomenclature for the chicken major histocompatibility B and Y complex. Immunogenetics. 564:261-79.

Moon, D.A., Veniamin, S.M., Parks-Dely, J.A. and Magor, K.F. 2005. The MHC of the Duck Anas platyrhynchos Contains Five ifferentially Expressed Class I Genes. The Journal of Immunology. 175: 6702–6712.

Mosmann, T.R. and Coffman, R.L. 1989. TH1 and TH2 cells: different patterns of lymphokine secretion lead to different functional properties. Annu. Rev. Immunol. 7: 145-173.

Nishibori. M,, Shimogiri, T., Hayashi, T. and Yasue, H. 2005. Molecular evidence for hybridization of species in the genus Gallus except for Gallus varius. Anim Genet. 36 (5) : 367-75.

Niu, D., Fu, Y., Luo, J., Ruan, H., Yu, X.P., Chen, G. and Zhang, Y.P. 2002. The origin and genetic diversity of Chinese native chicken breeds. Biochem Genet. 40 (5-6) : 163-74.

Okada I., Yamamoto Y., Hashiguchi T., Ito S. 1984. Phylogenetic studies on the Japanese native breeds of chickens, Jap. Poultry Sci. 21: 318–329.

Peters, 7.P., 1913. The cock. J. Amer. Oriental Soc. 33:363-401.

Peterson AT, Brisbin IL Jr. 1999. Genetic endangerment of wild red jungle fowl (Gallus gallus)? Bird Conservation International , 9:387-394.

Pharr,G.T., Bacon,L.D. and Dodgson,J.B. 1993. Analysis of B-L beta-chain gene expression in two chicken cDNA libraries. Immunogenetics 37 5, 381-385.

Plant, W.J., 1985. The Origin, Evolution, History and Distribution of the Domestic Fowl. Sapr'_-xto Part 2. Chicken Bone Recoveries. Privately published, 54 Bonar Street, Maitland N.S.W., Australia.

Pollard, J., 1977. Birds in Greek Life and Myth. Thames and Hudson, London.

Quinn TW and Wilson AC. 1993. Sequence Evolution in and Around the Ni itochondrial Control Region in Birds. J Mol Evol 37 : 417-425.

Ramirez V, Savoie P and Morais R. 1993. Molecular characterization of duck mitochondrial genome. J Mol Evol 37 : 296-310.

Randi E and Lucchini V. 1998. Organization and Evolution of the mitochondrial DNA Control Region in the Avian Genus Alectoris. J Mol Evol 47 : 449-462.

Roques S, Goddy JA, Negro JJ and Hiraldo F. 2004. Organization and Variation of the Mitochondrial Control Region in Two Vulture Species, Gypaetus barbatus abd Neophron percnopteus. J Heredity 95 : 332-337.

Saccone C, Gissi C, Lanave C, Larizza A, Pesole G and Reyes A. 2000. Evolution of the mitochondrial genetic system: an overview. Gene 261:153–159.

Saccone C, Pesole G and Sbisa E. 1991.The main regulatoru region of mammalian mitochondrial DNA : structure –function model and evolutionary pattern. J Mol Evol 33 : 83-91.

Sauer, C.O., 1969. Agricultural Origins and Dispersals. The Domestication of Animals and Foodstuffs, 2nd edition. M.I.T. Press, Cambridge, Massachusetts.

Sawai H, Kim HL, Kuno K, Suzuki S, Gotoh H, et al. 2010. The Origin and Genetic Variation of Domestic Chickens with Special Reference to Junglefowls Gallus g. gallus and G. varius. PLoS ONE 5(5): e10639. doi:10.1371/journal.pone.0010639

Sbisa E, Tanzarello F, Reyes A, Pesole G and Saccone C. 1997. Mammalian mitochondrial D-loop region structural analysis : identification of new conserved sequences and their functional and evolutionary implication. Gene 205 : 125-140.

Schierman, L.W. and Nordskog ,A. W. 1961.Relationship of blood type to histocompatibility in chickens. Science. 134:1008-1009.

Schmid,M., Nanda,I., Guttenbach,M., Steinlein, C., Hoehn, M., Schatr, M., Haaf, T., Weugend,S., Fries, R., Buerstedde, J.M., Wimmers, K., Burt, D.W., Smith, J. A., Hara,S., Law, A., Griffin, D.K., Bumstead, N., Kaufman, J., Thomson, P.A., Burke,T., Groenen, M.A., Crooijmans, R.P., Vignal, A., Fillon,V., Morisson,M., Pitel,F., Tixier-Boichard, M., Ladjali- Mohammedi, K., Hillel, J., Maki-Tanila,A., Cheng, H.H., Delany,M.E., Burnside, J., Mizuno,S. 2000. First report on chicken genes and chromosomes 2000, Cytogenet. Cell Genet., 90 : 169-218.

Schneider, K., Klaas, R., Kaspers, B. and Staeheli, P. 2001. Chicken interleukin-6 cDNA structure and biological properties. Eur. J. Biochem. 268, 4200-4206.

Sharma, Deepak. 2007. Final report on project entitled "Comparative genomic studies on wild and domesticated avian species". Submitted to DBT, New Delhi

Shaw I., Powell, T.J., Marston, D.A., Baker, K., Hateren, A., Riegert, P., Wiles, M.V., Milne, S., Beck, S. and Kaufman, J. 2007. Different evolutionary histories of the two classical class I genes BF1 and BF2 illustrate drift and selection within the stable MHC haplotypes of chickens. The Journal of Immunology, 2007, 178: 5744-5752

Shaw, G. and Kamen, R. 1986. A conserved AU sequence from the 3′ untranslated region of GM-CSF mRNA mediates selective mRNA degradation. *Cell* 46, 659-67.

Shiina,T., Oka,A., Imanishi,T., Hanzawa,K., Gojobori,T., Watanabe,S. and Inoko,H. 1999. Multiple class I loci expressed by the quail MhC. Immunogenetics 49 5, 456-460.

Shukla, S.K. 2010. Genetic polymorphism in BF region in Red Jungle Fowl and domestic chicken Submitted to Bundelkhand University, Jhansi.

Singh Anup, , Gupta J., Churchil RR, Sharma Deepak and Singh RV. 2007. Genetic diversity between Red Jungle Fowl and domestic chicken for BLB2 region. J Appl. Anim. Res. 31 : 69-72.

Singh, S.K. 2009. Genetic polymorphism in BLB2 region and its association with immunocompetence and production traits in guinea fowl Numida meleagris. PhD thesis, Submitted to BU,Jhansi.

Sreekumar, E., Premraj, A., and Rasool, T.J. 2005. Duck Anas platyrhynchos, Japanese quail Coturnix coturnix japonica and other avian interleukin-2 reveals significant conservation of gene organization, promoter elements and functional residues. Inter. J. Immunogenetics 32, 355–365

Stevens, L. & Duncan, D. 1988. Peptied mapping of ovoglobulins G2A and G2B in the domestic fowl. British poultry Science, 29, 665-9

Sugano, S., Stoeckle, M.Y.and Hanafusa, H., 1987. Transformation by Rous sarcoma virus induces a novel gene with homology to a mitogenic platelet protein. Cell 49, 321–328.

Taran, M., 1975. Early records of the domestic fowl in ancient Judea. Ibis 117:109-110.

Tegetmeier, W.B., 1867. The Poultry book : Comprising the Breeding and Management of Profitable and Ornamental Poultry, Their Qualities and George Characteristics. George Routledge and Sons, London.

Tomar, A., Shukla, P.K., Gupta, J., Singh, A., Churchil, R.R. and Sharma D (2007). Genetic polymorphism among red jungle fowl and domesticated chicken detected by DNA markers. J. Appl. Anim Res. 31 : 205-208.

Wallny., H. J,. Avila, D., Hunt, L.G. .2006. Peptide motifs of the single dominantly expressed cl.ass I molecule explain the striking MHC-determined response to Rous sarcoma virus in chickens. Proc. Natl. Acad. Sci. U S A. 103,1434–1439.

Watson, W., 1969. Early animal domestication in China. In: Ucko, P.J., and G.W. Dimbleby, editors. The Domestication and EzpPoitacian of Plants andAnimals.Aldine Publishing Co., Chicago.

Weining, K. C., Sick, C., Kaspers, B. and Staeheli, P. 1998. A chicken homolog of mammalian interleukin-1b: cDNA cloning and purification of active recombinant protein. Eur. J. Biochem. 258, 994–1000.

Weiss, R.A., and P.M. Biggs, 1972 Leukosis and Marek's disease viruses of feral red jungle fowl and domestic fowl in Malaya. J. Natl.Cancer Inst. 49:1713-1725.

West, B., and B.-X Zhou, 1988. Did chickens go north? New evidence for domestication. J. Archaeol. Sci. 15:515-533.

Wittzell,H., Bernot,A., Auffray,C. and Zoorob,R.1999. Concerted evolution of two Mhc class II B loci in pheasants and domestic chickens. Mol. Biol. Evol. 16 4: 479-90.

Wood-Gush, D.G.M., 1959. A history of the domestic chicken from antiquity to the 19th century. Poultry Sci. 38:321-326.

Wood-Gush, D.G.M., 1985. Domestication. In: Campbell, B., and E. Lack, editors. A Dictionary of Birds. T. & A.D. Poyser, Calton, Staffordshire.

Wu, Y. F., Liu, H. J., Chiou, S. H. and Lee, L. H. 2007. Sequence and phylogenetic analysis of interleukin IL-1b-encoding genes of five avian species and structural and functional homology among these IL-1b proteins. Vet. Immunol. Immunopathol. 116, 37–46.

Xia, C., Lin, C.Y., Xu, G.X., Hu, T.J. and Yang, T.Y. 2004. cDNA cloning and genomic structure of the duck Anas platyrhynchos MHC class I gene. Immunogenetics. 56 : 304-309.

Yan, R.Q., Li, X.S., Yang, T.Y. and Xia, C. 2005a. Characterization of BF2 and B2m in three Chinese chicken lines. Veterinary Immunology and Immunopathology. 108 : 417-425.

Yan, R.Q., Li, X.S., Yang, T.Y. and Xia, C. 2005b. Structures and homology modeling of chicken major histocompatibility complex protein class I BF2 and beta2m. Mol Immuunology 43 : 1040-46.

Zeuner, F.E., 1963. A History of Domesticated Animals. Hutchinson & Co., London.

Zhou, J.Y., Chen, J.G., Wang, J.Y. and Kwang, J. 2003. Cloning and genetic evolution analysis of chIl-2 gene of Chinese local breeds, Prog. Biochem. Biophys. 30 384-389.

Zoorob, R., Behar, G., Kroemer, G. and Auffray, C., 1990.Organisation of a functional chicken class II gene. Immunogenetics 31:179-187.

Zoorob, R., Bernot, A., Renoir, A.D.M., Choukri, F. and Auffray, C. 1993. Chicken MHC class II b genes, analysis of interallelic and intralocus sequence variance. Eur. J. Immunol. 23: 1139-1195.

□□□